KEEP IT PLANT-BASED

The Cookbook With Over 50 Whole Food, Plant-Based Recipes That Can Be Made With Fewer Ingredients From Breakfast Through Dessert.

Botanika Green Way

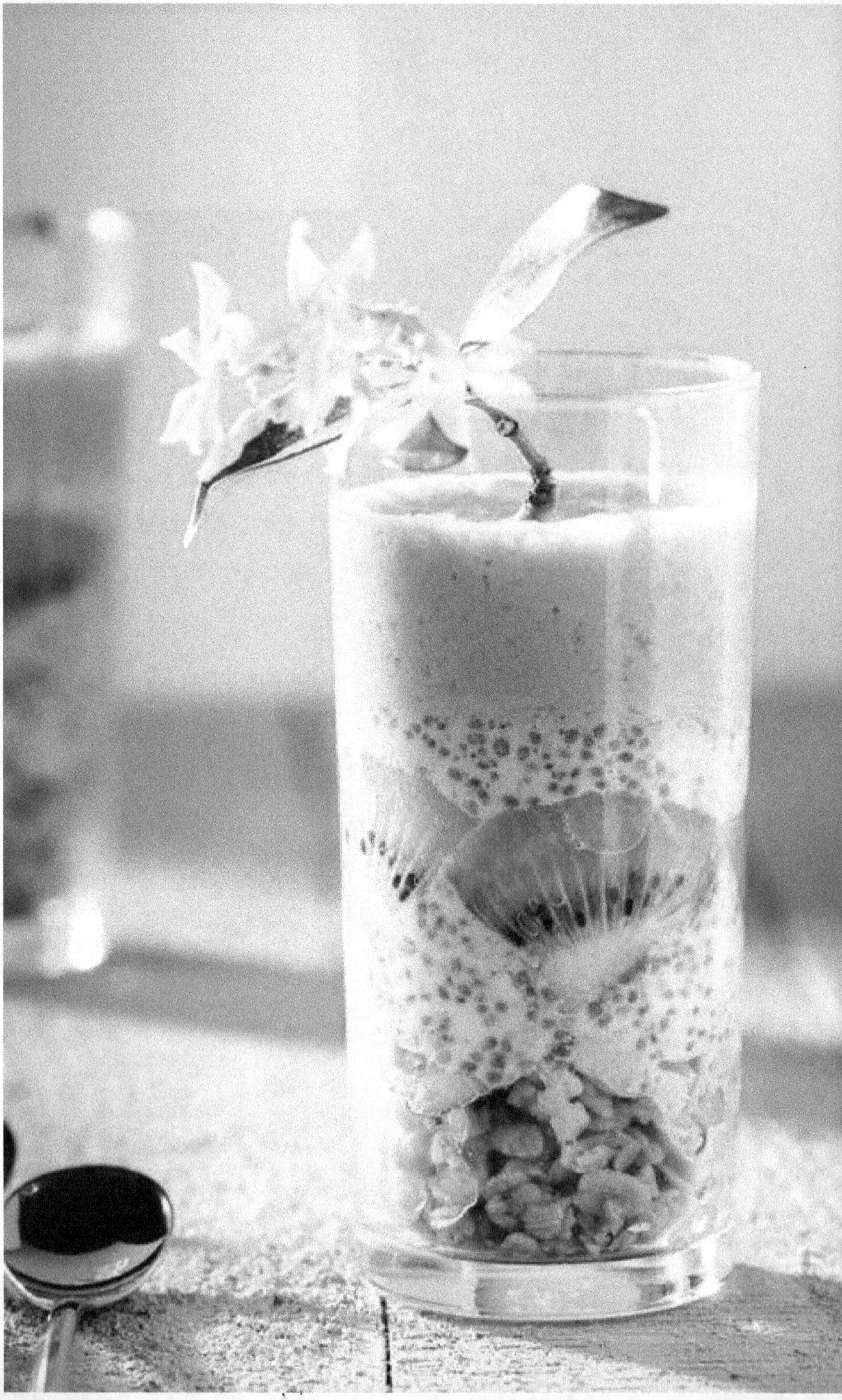

liable for any hardship or damages that may befall them after undertaking the information described herein.

Additionally, the information in the following pages is intended only for informational purposes and should thus be thought of as universal. As befitting its nature, it is presented without assurance regarding its prolonged validity or interim quality. Trademarks that are mentioned are done without written consent and can in no way be considered an endorsement from the trademark holder.

Table of Contents

INTRODUCTION

A plant-based diet is a diet based primarily on whole plant foods. Hence, it excludes animal-sourced foods, hydrogenated oils, refined sugars, and processed foods. A whole food plant-based diet does not consist solely of fruits and vegetables. It includes unprocessed or barely processed oils with healthy fats like extra-virgin olive oil, whole grains, legumes, seeds, and nuts, as well as herbs and spices.

What is the Plant-Based Diet?

The plant-based diet may seem similar to a vegetarian or vegan diet, but it is neither. It's not a diet but a healthy lifestyle. It uses food from plants, and it excludes processed foods like white rice and added sugars, which are allowed in vegan and vegetarian diets.

A plant-based diet is not a diet; it's a healthy way of life

The secret to a healthy diet is simpler than you ever thought! When following a plant-based dietary regimen, you should focus on plant-based foods and avoid animal-sourced food. Whether you are already following a vegan diet or are considering trying this lifestyle, this plant-based, budget-friendly food list makes your grocery shopping easy to manage.

- **VEGETABLES**

Try to include different types of vegetables in your diet from above-ground vegetables to root vegetables, which grow underground.

- **FRUITS**

Choose affordable fruits that are in season. Add frozen fruit to your grocery list since they are just as nutritious as fresh produce. They can be used in smoothies, toppings, compotes, or preserves. On the other hand, dried fruit generally contains a lot of antioxidants, especially polyphenols. It has been proven that eating dried fruits can prevent heart disease and some types of cancer.

- **NUTS & SEEDS**

Nuts and seeds offer different dietary benefits. They do not only ensure essential nutrients but are also offer a variety of flavors. This "ready to eat" food is a perfect snack with dried fruits and trail mix, essential vegan foods to stockpile for an emergency.

- **RICE & GRAINS**

Rice and grains are versatile and easy to incorporate into your diet. Leftovers reheat wonderfully and can be served at any time of the day, turning simple and inexpensive ingredients into a full-fledged meal. You can also make healthy nut butters such as tahini or peanut butter.

- **BEANS & LEGUMES**

Legumes and beans are highly affordable, and there's no end to the variety of tasty dishes you can cook with them. These humble but powerful foods are packed with vitamins, minerals, protein, and dietary fiber. In addition to being super-healthy and versatile, legumes pair very well with other proteins, vegetables, and grains.

- **HEALTHY FATS**

Don't underestimate the importance of quality fats in cooking. Coconut oil, olive oil, and avocado are always good to have on hand.

- **NON-DAIRY PRODUCTS**

Using a plant-based cheese or milk lends flavor, texture, and nutrition to your meals. You can find fantastic products on the market, and this book has many wonderful recipes for feta, vegan ricotta, and plant-based milk.

- **HERBS, SPICES & CONDIMENTS**

A handful of fresh herbs will add that little something extra to your soups, stews, dips, or casseroles. Condiments such as mustard, ketchup, vegan mayonnaise, and plant-based sauces can be used in salads, casseroles, and spreads. Choosing their distinctive flavors to complement vegetables, grains and legumes will help you to make the most of your vegan dishes. Herbs and spices are naturally plant-based, but play it safe and look for a label that says *Vegan-friendly*.

- **BAKING GOODS & CANNED GOODS**

These vegan essentials include all types of flour, baking powder, baking soda, and yeast. Further, cocoa powder, vegan chocolate, and sweeteners are good to have on hand. As for the healthy vegan sweeteners, opt for fresh or dried fruits, agave syrup, maple syrup, and stevia. When it comes to canned goods, stock your pantry with cooking essentials such as tomato, sauerkraut, pickles, low sodium chickpeas and beans, coconut milk, green chilies, pumpkin puree, tomato sauce, low sodium corn, and artichoke hearts. Thus, if you want to make sure you have nutritious, delicious, and quality meals for you and your family, having a vegan pantry is halfway there.

Why You Ought to Reduce Your Intake of Processed and Animal-Based Foods

You have heard over and over that processed food has adverse effects on your health. You might have also been told repeatedly to stay away from foods with lots of preservatives. However, you may have never heard any genuine or concrete facts about why these foods are unsafe. Consequently, let us properly dissect it to help you properly comprehend why you ought to stay away from these offenders.

- **They have massive habit-forming characteristics**

Humans have a predisposition toward being addicted to some specific foods; however, the reality is that the fault is not wholly ours.

Every one of the unhealthy treats we relish now and then triggers a dopamine release. This creates a pleasurable effect in our brain, but the excitement is usually short-lived. The discharged dopamine gradually causes an attachment, and this is the reason some people consistently go back to eat certain unhealthy foods even when they know they're unhealthy and unnecessary. You can get rid of this by avoiding the temptation completely.

- **They are sugar-laden and heavy in glucose-fructose syrup**

Animal-based and processed foods are laden with refined sugars and glucose-fructose syrup, which has almost no nutritional value. An ever-increasing number of studies are affirming what several people presumed from the start: that genetically modified foods bring about inflammatory bowel disease, which consequently makes it increasingly difficult for the body to assimilate essential nutrients. The disadvantages that result from your body being unable to assimilate essential nutrients from consumed foods rightly cannot be overemphasized.

Processed and animal-based food products contain plenteous amounts of refined carbohydrates. Indeed, your body requires carbohydrates to give it energy to function.

In any case, refining carbs dispenses with the fundamental supplements in the way that refining entire grains disposes of the whole grain part. What remains in the wake of refining is what's considered empty carbs or empty calories. These can negatively affect the metabolic system in your body by sharply increasing your blood sugar and insulin levels.

- **They contain lots of synthetic ingredients**

When your body takes in non-natural ingredients, it regards them as of foreign substance and a health threat. It isn't accustomed to identifying synthetic compounds like sucralose or synthesized sugars. Hence, in defense of your health against this foreign "aggressor," your body does what it's programmed to do to safeguard your health: It sets off an immune reaction to tackle this "enemy" compound, which indirectly weakens your body's general disease alertness, making you susceptible to illnesses. The energy expended by your body in triggering your immune system could be better utilized somewhere else.

- **They contain constituent elements that set off a sensation in your body**

A part of processed and animal-based foods contains compounds like glucose-fructose syrup, monosodium glutamate, and specific food dyes that can trigger some addictions. They teach your body to receive a benefit whenever you consume them. Monosodium glutamate, for example, is added to many store-bought baked foods. This additive slowly conditions your palate to relish and crave the taste.

- **This reward-centric arrangement makes you crave it increasingly, which ends up exposing you to the danger of over-consuming calories**

For animal protein, usually, the expression "subpar" is used to allude to plant proteins since they generally have lower levels of essential amino acids as against animal-sourced protein. Nevertheless, what the vast majority don't know is that large amounts of essential amino acids can prove detrimental to your health. Let me break it down further for you.

- **Animal-sourced protein has no fiber**

In their pursuit to consume animal protein, the vast majority wind up dislodging the plant protein that was previously available in their body. Replacing the plant proteins with its animal variant is harmful because, in contrast to plant protein, animal proteins typically are deficient in fiber, phyto-nutrients, and antioxidant properties. Fiber insufficiency is a regular feature across various regions and societies on the planet. In America, for example, according to the National Academy of Medicine, the typical adult takes in roughly 15 grams of dietary fiber daily rather than the recommended daily quantity of 25 to 30 grams. A deficiency in dietary fiber often leads to a heightened risk of breast and colorectal cancers, in addition to constipation, inflammatory bowel disease, and cardiovascular disease.

- **Animal protein brings about an upsurge in phosphorus levels in the body**

Animal protein has significant levels of phosphorus. Our bodies stabilize these plenteous amounts of phosphorus by producing and discharging a hormone known as fibroblast growth factor 23 (FGF23). Studies have shown that this hormone is dangerous to our veins. FGF23 also causes asymmetrical expansion of heart muscles—a determinant for congestive heart failure and even mortality in some advanced cases.

Having discussed the many problems associated with animal protein, it becomes more apt to replace its "high quality" perception with the tag "highly hazardous." In contrast to caffeine, which has a withdrawal effect if it's discontinued abruptly, you can stop taking processed and animal-based foods right away without any withdrawals. Possibly the only thing that you'll give up is the ease of some meals taking little to no time to prepare.

Health Benefits of the Plant-Based Diet

Plant-based eating is one of the healthiest diets in the world. It should include plenty of fresh products, whole grains, legumes, and healthy fats such as seeds and nuts, which are rich in antioxidants, minerals, vitamins, and dietary fiber.

Scientific research has shown that higher use of plant-based foods is connected to a lower risk of death from conditions such as cardiovascular disease, diabetes, hypertension, and obesity. Vegan eating relies heavily on healthy staples, avoiding animal products. Animal products contain much more fat than plant-based foods; it's not a shocker that studies have shown that meat-eaters have nine times the obesity rate of vegans.

This leads us to the next point, one of the greatest benefits of the vegan diet: weight loss. While many people choose to live a vegan life for ethical reasons, the diet itself can help you achieve your weight loss goals. If you're struggling to shift pounds, you may want to consider trying a plant-based diet. How exactly? As a vegan, you will reduce the number of high-calorie foods such as full-fat dairy products, fatty fish, pork, and other cholesterol-containing foods such as eggs. Try replacing such foods with high-fiber and protein-rich alternatives that will keep you fuller longer. The key is focusing on nutrient-dense, clean and natural foods and avoiding empty calories such as sugar, saturated fats, and highly processed foods. Here are a few tricks that help me maintain my weight on the vegan diet. I eat vegetables as a main course; I consume good fats in moderation (good fats such as olive oil do not make you fat); I exercise regularly and cook at home. Plant foods are an excellent source of many nutrients that boost the body's metabolism in many ways. They are easy to digest thanks to their rich content of antioxidants.

- **Reduced Risk of Heart Diseases**

Processed and animal foods are responsible for much heart disease. A whole foods plant-based diet is better at nourishing the body with essential nutrients while improving the heart's function to produce and transport blood to and from the various body parts.

- **Prevents and Heals Diabetes**

Plant-based foods are excellent at reducing high blood sugar. Many studies comparing a vegetarian and vegan diet to a regular meat-filled diet proved that dieting with more plant foods reduced the risk of diabetes by 50 percent.

- **Improved Cognitive Incline**

Fruits and vegetables are excellent for cleansing and boosting metabolism. They release high numbers of plant compounds and antioxidants that slow or prevent cognitive decline. On a plant-based diet, the brain is boosted with sustainable energy, promoting sharp memory, language, thinking, and judgment abilities.

- **Quick Weight Loss**

A high animal food diet is known to drive weight gain. Switching to a plant-based diet helps the body shed fat walls easily, which quickly drives weight loss.

BREAKFAST

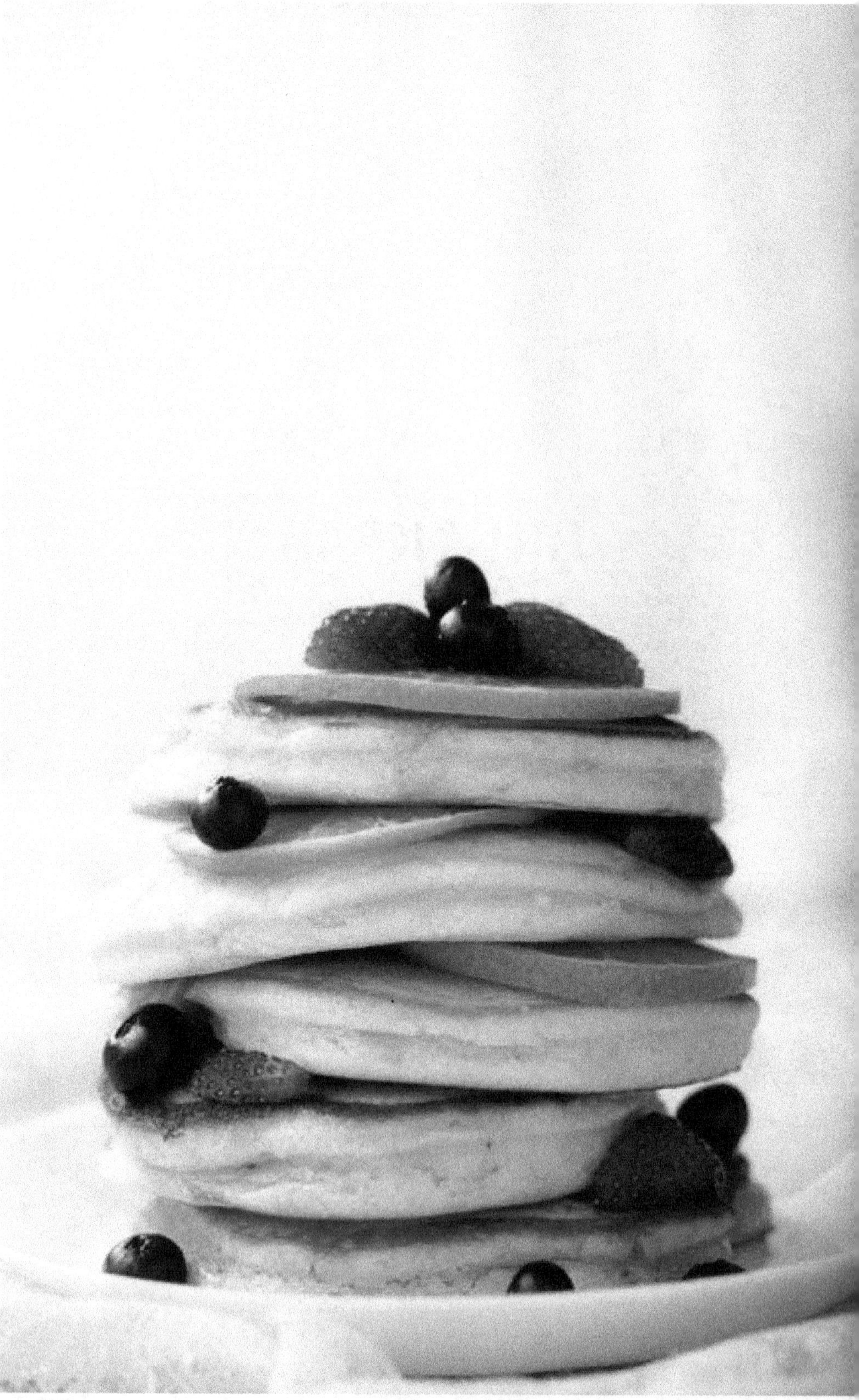

Almond Oatmeal Porridge

6 Servings

Preparation Time: 25 minutes

Ingredients

- 2 ½ cups Vegetable broth
- 1 tbsp Pearl barley
- ½ cup slivered Almonds
- ¼ cup nutritional Yeast
- 2 cups old-fashioned Rolled oats
- 2 ½ cups almond Milk
- ½ cup steel-cut Oats

Directions

- Add the broth and almond milk in a pot over medium heat and bring to a boil.

- Stir in oats, pearl barley, almond slivers, and nutritional yeast. Reduce the heat and simmer for 20 minutes.

- Add in the rolled oats; cook for an additional 5 minutes until creamy. Allow cooling before serving.

Blackberry Waffles

6 Servings

Preparation Time: 15 minutes

Ingredients

- 1 ½ cups Whole-wheat flour
- ½ tsp Salt
- 1 tsp ground Cinnamon
- 2 cups Soy milk
- 1 tbsp fresh Lemon juice
- 1 tsp Lemon zest
- ¼ cup Plant butter, melted
- ½ cup fresh Blackberries
- ½ cup old-fashioned Oats
- ¼ cup Date sugar
- 3 tsps Baking powder

Directions

- Preheat the waffle iron.

- In a bowl, mix flour, oats, sugar, baking powder, salt, and cinnamon. Set aside.

- In another bowl, mix milk, lemon juice, lemon zest, and butter. Add into the wet ingredients and whisk to combine.

- Add the batter to the hot greased waffle iron, using approximately a ladleful for each waffle. Cook for 3-5 minutes, until golden brown.

- Repeat the process until no batter is left. Serve topped with blackberries.

Classic Walnut Waffles with Maple Syrup

6 Servings

Preparation Time: 15 minutes

Ingredients

- 1 ¾ cups Whole-wheat flour
- 1 ½ cups Soy milk
- 3 tbsps pure Maple syrup
- 3 tbsps Plant butter, melted
- ⅓ cup Coarsely ground walnuts
- 1 tbsp Baking powder

Directions

- Preheat the waffle iron and grease with oil.

- Mix the flour, walnuts, baking powder, and salt in a bowl. Set aside.

- In another bowl, mix the milk and butter.

- Add into the walnut mixture and whisk until well combined. Spoon a ladleful of the batter onto the waffle iron.

- Cook for 3-5 minutes, until golden brown.

- Repeat the process until no batter is left. Top with maple syrup to serve.

Orange-Bran Cups with Dates

8 Servings

Preparation Time: 30 minutes

Ingredients

- 1 tsp Vegetable oil
- ½ cup Dates, chopped
- 3 tsps Baking powder
- ½ tsp ground Cinnamon
- ½ tsp Salt
- ⅓ cup Brown sugar
- ¾ cup fresh Orange juice
- 3 cups Bran flakes cereal
- 1 ½ cups Whole-wheat flour

Directions

- Preheat oven to 400°F. Grease a 12-cup muffin tin with oil.

- Mix the bran flakes, flour, dates, baking powder, cinnamon, and salt in a bowl.

- In another bowl, mix the sugar and orange juice until blended.

- Pour into the dry mixture and whisk.

- Divide the mixture between the cups of the muffin tin. Bake for 20 minutes or until golden brown and set.

- Cool for a few minutes before removing from the tin and serve.

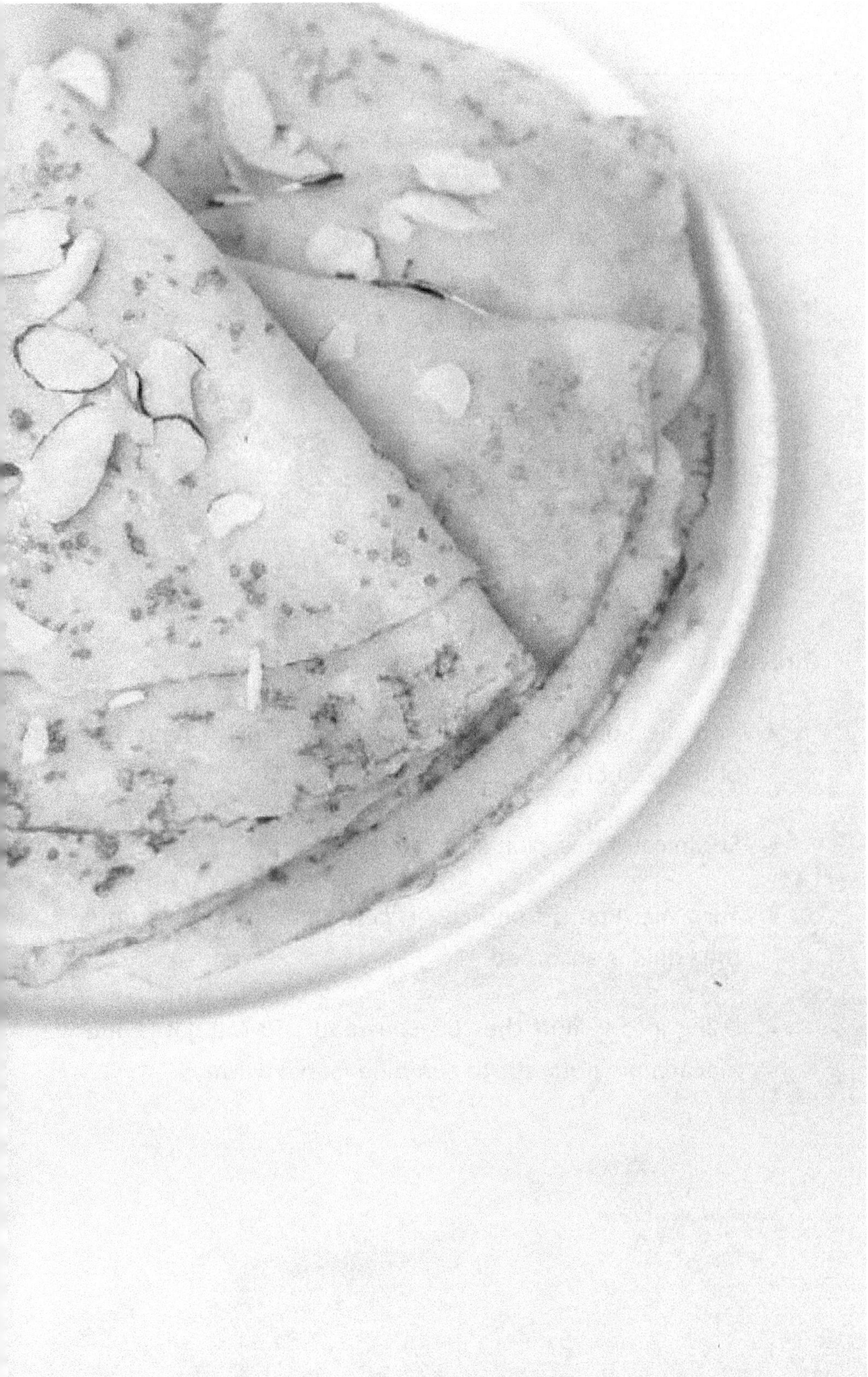

Apple-Date Couscous with Macadamia Nuts

6 Servings

Preparation Time: 20 minutes

Ingredients

- 3 cups Apple juice
- 1 tsp ground Cinnamon
- ¼ tsp ground Cloves
- ½ cup Dried dates
- ½ cup chopped Macadamia nuts
- 1 ½ cups couscous

Directions

- Add the apple juice into a pot over medium heat and bring to a boil.

- Stir in couscous, cinnamon, and cloves.

- Turn the heat off and cover. Let sit for 5 minutes until the liquid is absorbed.

- Using a fork, fluff the couscous and add the dates and macadamia nuts, stir to combine. Serve warm.

Carrot-Strawberry Smoothie

4 Servings

Preparation Time: 5 minutes

Ingredients

- 1 cup peeled and diced Carrots
- 1 Apple, chopped
- 2 tbsps Maple syrup
- 2 cups unsweetened Almond milk
- 1 cup Strawberries

Directions

- Put all the ingredients in a blender. Blend until smooth.

- Pour in glasses and serve.

DRINKS

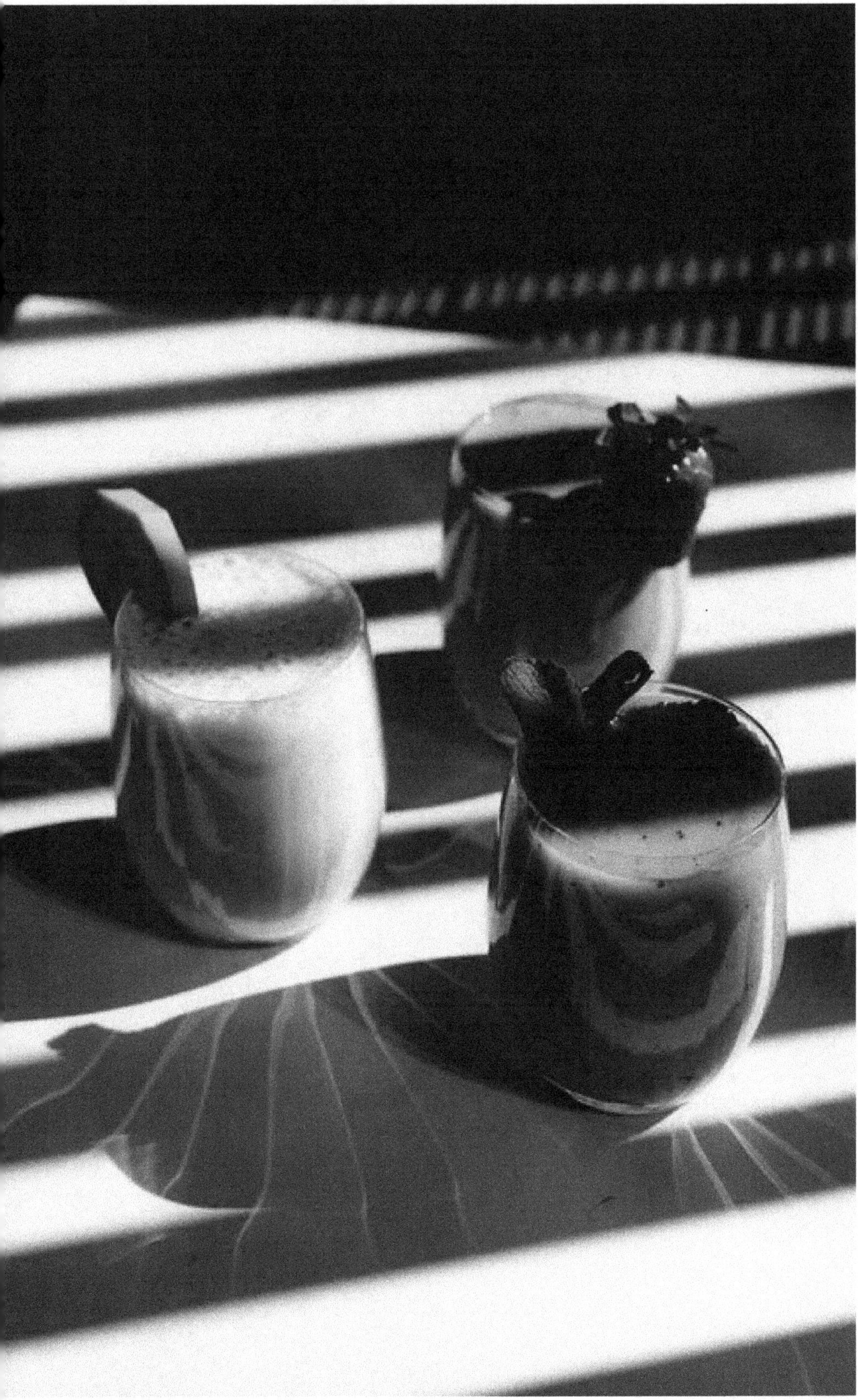

Chai and Chocolate Milkshake

2 Servings

Preparation Time: 5 minutes

Ingredients

- 1 and ½ cups of almond milk, sweetened or unsweetened
- 3 bananas, peeled and frozen 12 hours before use
- 4 dates, pitted
- 1 and ½ teaspoons of chocolate powder, sweetened or unsweetened
- ½ teaspoon of vanilla extract
- ½ teaspoon of cinnamon
- ¼ teaspoon of ground ginger
- Pinch of ground cardamom
- Pinch of ground cloves
- Pinch of ground nutmeg
- ½ cup of ice cubes

Directions

- Add all the ingredients to a blender except for the ice-cubes. Pulse until smooth and creamy, add the ice-cubes, pulse a few more times and serve.

Soothing Ginger Tea Drink

8 Servings

Preparation Time: 5 minutes

Ingredients

- 1 tablespoon of minced ginger root
- 2 tablespoons of honey
- 15 green tea bags
- 32 fluid ounce of white grape juice
- 2 quarts of boiling water

Directions

- Pour water into a 4-quarts slow cooker, immerse tea bags, cover the cooker, and let stand for 10 minutes.
- After 10 minutes, remove and discard tea bags and stir in the remaining ingredients.
- Return cover to the slow cooker, let cook at high heat setting for 2 hours or until heated through.
- When done, strain the liquid and serve hot or cold.

Ginger Cherry Cider

16 Servings

Preparation Time: 1 hour 5 minutes

Ingredients

- 2 knobs of ginger, each about 2 inches
- 6-ounce of cherry gelatin
- 4 quarts of apple cider

Direction

- Using a 6-quarts slow cooker, pour the apple cider and add the ginger.
- Stir, and then cover the slow cooker with its lid. Let it cook for 3 hours at the high heat setting or until it is heated thoroughly.
- Then add and stir the gelatin properly, then continue cooking for another hour.
- When done, remove the ginger and serve the drink hot or cold.

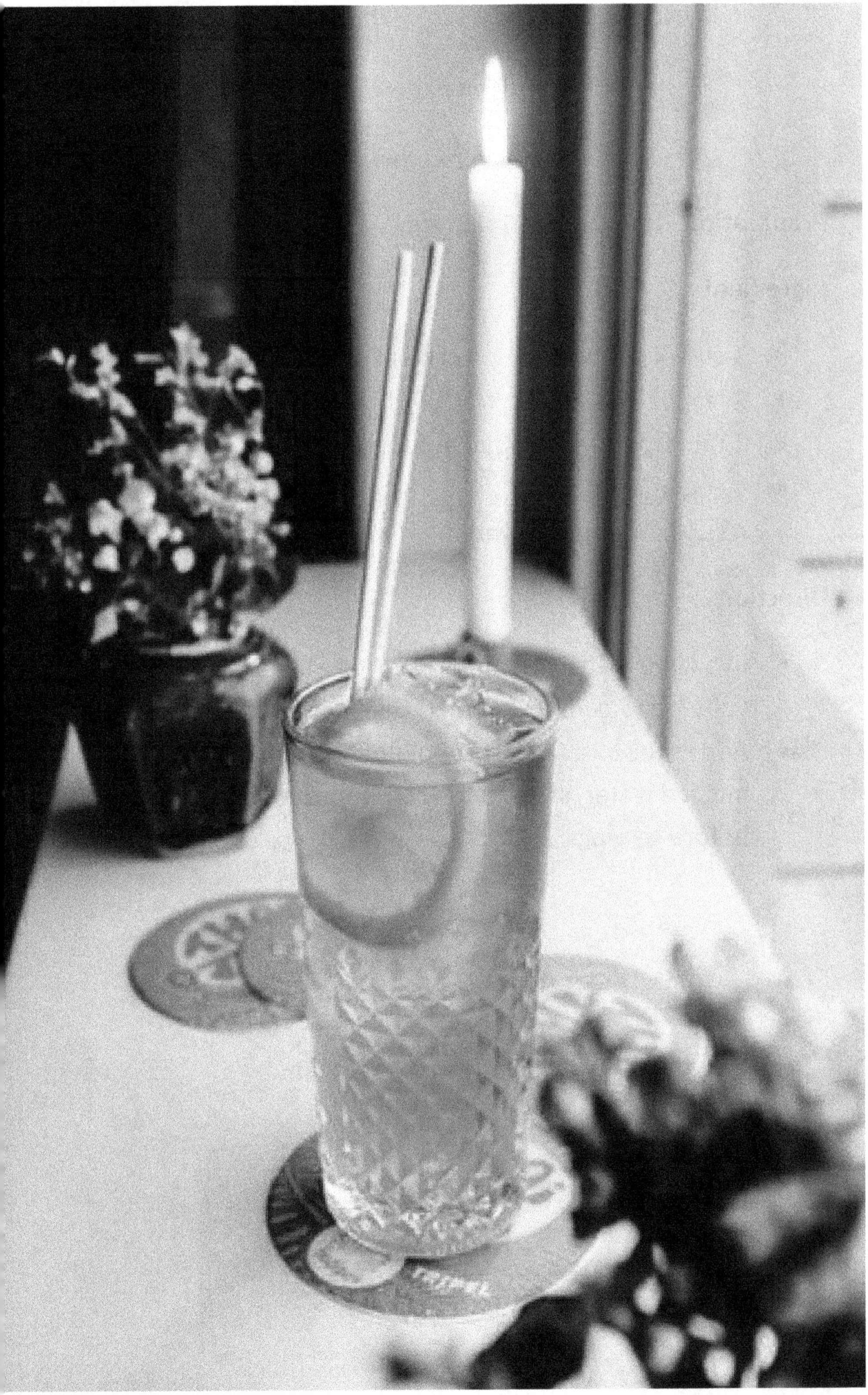

Colorful Infused Water

8 Servings

Preparation Time: 1 hour 5 minutes

Ingredients

- 1 cup of strawberries, fresh or frozen
- 1 cup of blueberries, fresh or frozen
- 1 tablespoon of baobab powder
- 1 cup of ice cubes
- 4 cups of sparkling water

Directions

- In a large water jug, add in the sparkling water, ice cubes, and baobab powder. Give it a good stir.
- Add in the strawberries and blueberries and cover the infused water, store in the refrigerator for one hour before serving.

LUNCH

Watercress & Mushroom Spaghetti

6 Servings

Preparation Time: 30 minutes

Ingredients

- 1 lb whole-wheat spaghetti
- 1 tbsp sake
- 3 tbsps soy sauce
- 1 tsp hot sauce
- A handful of watercress
- ¼ cup chopped fresh parsley
- Black pepper to taste
- 3 tbsps plant butter
- 2 tbsps olive oil
- 2 shallots, finely chopped
- 2 garlic cloves, minced
- ½ lb chopped button mushrooms

Directions

- Cook spaghetti in lightly salted water in a large pot over medium heat until al dente, 10 minutes.

- Drain and set aside. Heat butter and olive oil in a skillet and sauté shallots, garlic, and mushrooms for 5 minutes. Stir in sake, soy sauce, and hot sauce.

- Cook for 1 minute. Toss spaghetti in the sauce along with watercress and parsley.

- Season with black pepper. Dish the food and serve warm.

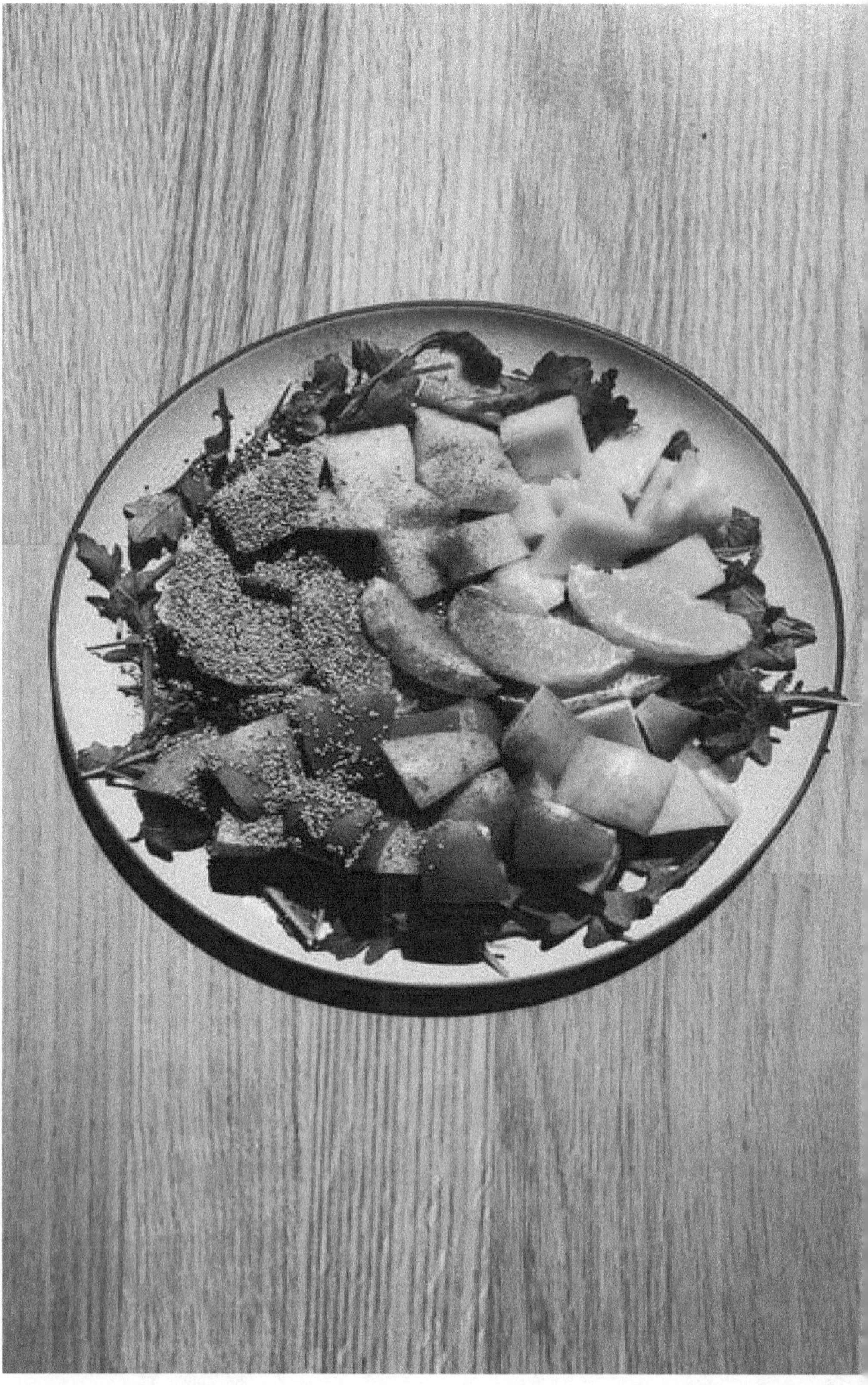

Rice with Green Lentil & Celery

6 Servings

Preparation Time: 50 minutes

Ingredients

- 2 tbsps olive oil
- 4 garlic cloves, minced
- 3 cups vegetable broth
- 1 tsp oregano
- 1 cup green lentils, rinsed
- ¼ cup chopped tomatoes
- 1 lime, juiced
- 1 cup brown rice
- 1 lb tempeh, cut into cubes
- 1 yellow onion, chopped
- Salt and black pepper to taste
- 1 tsp chili powder
- 1 tsp cumin powder
- 2 celery stalks, chopped
- 2 carrots diced

Directions

- Heat the olive oil in a large pot, season the tempeh with salt, pepper, and cook for 10 minutes.

- Stir in chili powder, cumin powder, onion, celery, carrots, garlic, and cook for 5 minutes.

- Pour in vegetable broth, oregano, green lentils, tomatoes, brown rice, and green chilies. Cover the pot and cook for 18-20 minutes.

- Open the lid, adjust the taste with salt, black pepper, and mix in the lime juice. Serve.

Spinach & Chickpea Pizza with Avocado

6 Servings

Preparation Time: 40 minutes

Ingredients

- 3 tbsps olive oil
- 1 cup red pizza sauce
- 1 cup baby spinach
- 1 (15 oz) can chickpeas, drained
- 1 avocado, chopped
- ¼ cup grated plant-based Parmesan
- 1 tsp oregano
- 3 ½ cups whole-wheat flour
- 1 tsp yeast
- 1 tsp salt
- 1 pinch sugar

Directions

- Preheat the oven the 350 F and lightly grease a pizza pan with cooking spray.

- In a bowl, mix flour, nutritional yeast, salt, sugar, olive oil, and 1 cup of warm water until smooth dough forms.

- Allow rising for an hour or until the dough doubles in size. Spread the dough on the pizza pan and apply the pizza sauce on top.

- Top with oregano, baby spinach, chickpeas, avocado, and plant Parmesan cheese. Bake for 20 minutes or until the cheese melts.

- Remove from the oven, cool for 5 minutes, slice, and serve.

Herby Quinoa with Walnuts

6 Servings

Preparation Time: 20 minutes

Ingredients

- 1 cup quinoa, well-rinsed
- 2 tbsps finely chopped basil
- 2 tbsps finely chopped mint
- 2 tbsps chopped sundried tomatoes
- 1 tbsp olive oil
- ½ tsp lemon zest
- 1 tbsp fresh lemon juice
- 2 tbsps minced walnuts
- 2 cups vegetable broth
- 2 garlic cloves, minced, divided
- ¼ cup chopped chives
- 2 tbsps finely chopped parsley

Directions

- In a pot, combine quinoa, vegetable broth, and garlic.

- Boil until the quinoa is tender and the liquid absorbs for 10-15 minutes.

- Fluff with a fork and stir in chives, parsley, basil, mint, tomatoes, olive oil, zest, lemon juice, and walnuts. Warm for 5 minutes. Serve.

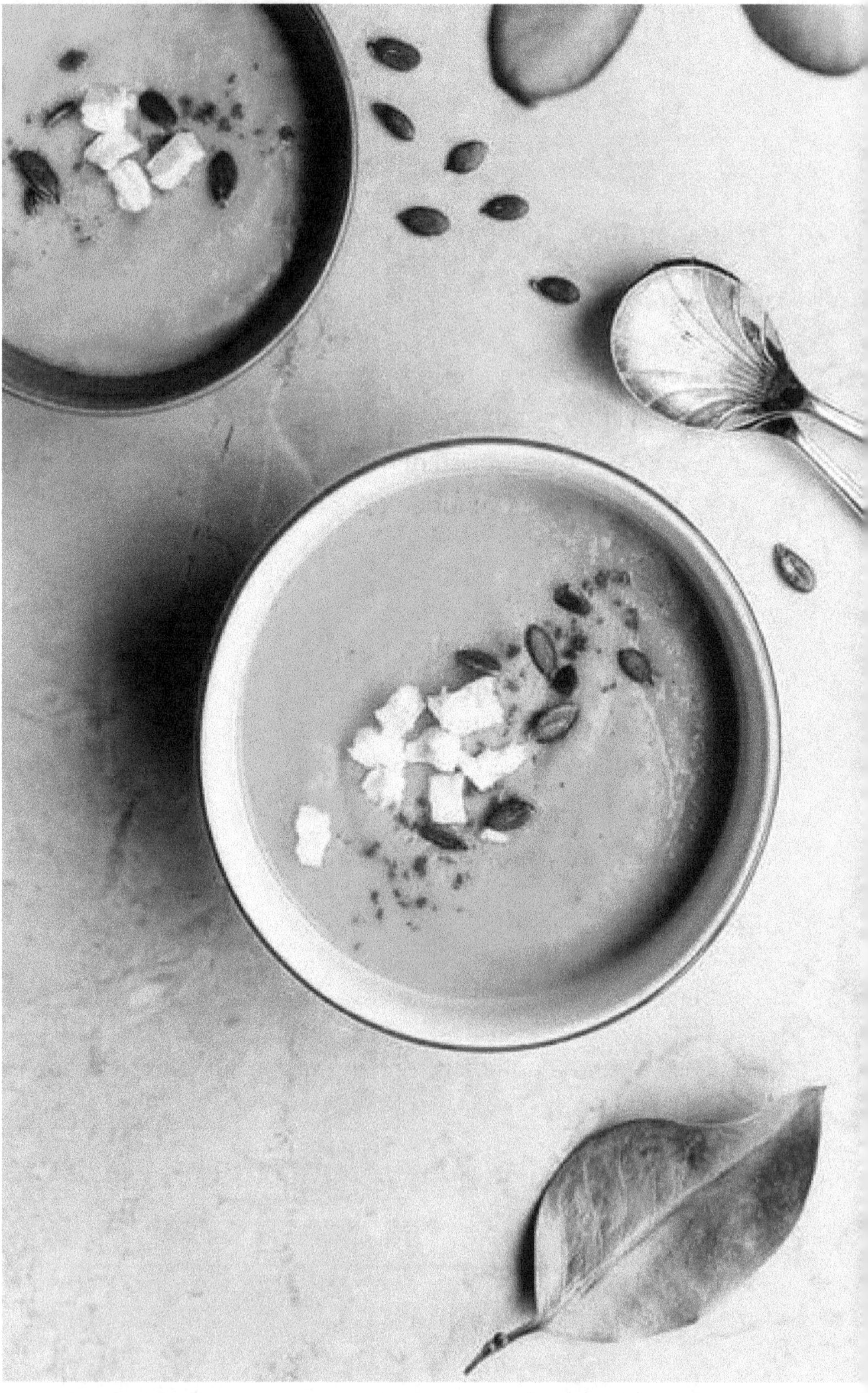

Pasta Primavera with Cherry Tomatoes

6 Servings

Preparation Time: 25 minutes

Ingredients

- 2 tbsps olive oil
- 1 cup dry white wine
- Salt and black pepper to taste
- 2 cups cherry tomatoes, halved
- 3 tbsps plant butter, cubed
- 1 lemon, zested and juiced
- 1 cup packed fresh basil leaves
- 8 oz whole-wheat feedline pasta
- ½ tsp paprika
- 1 small red onion, sliced
- 2 garlic cloves, minced

Directions

- Heat olive oil in a pot and mix in feedline, paprika, onion, garlic, and stir-fry for 2-3 minutes.

- Mix in white wine, salt, and pepper. Cover with water. Cook until the water absorbs and the feedline al dente, 5 minutes.

- Mix in the cherry tomatoes, butter, lemon zest, lemon juice, and basil leaves. Serve warm.

Cherry & Quinoa Tacos

6 Servings

Preparation Time: 25 minutes

Ingredients

- ½ cup brown quinoa
- 2 tsps olive oil
- 1 ½ cups shredded carrots
- 1 ¼ cups fresh cherries, halved
- 2 tbsps soy sauce
- 1 tbsp pure maple syrup
- 4 (8-inch) tortilla wraps
- 4 scallions, chopped
- 2 tbsps plain vinegar

Directions

- Cook the quinoa in 1 cup of slightly salted water in a pot for 15 minutes. Fluff and set aside.

- Heat olive oil in a skillet and sauté carrots, cherries, and scallions. In a small bowl, mix vinegar, soy sauce, and maple syrup

- . Stir the mixture into the vegetable mixture. Simmer for 5 minutes.

- Spread the tortillas on a flat surface, spoon the mixture at the center, fold the sides and ends to wrap in the filling. Serve.

Quinoa a la Puttanesca

6 Servings

Preparation Time: 30 minutes

Ingredients

- 1 cup brown quinoa
- 2 garlic cloves, minced
- 1 tbsp olive oil
- 1 tbsp chopped fresh parsley
- ¼ cup chopped fresh basil
- 1/8 tsp red chili flakes
- 2 cups water
- 1/8 tsp salt
- 4 cups plum tomatoes, chopped
- 4 pitted green olives, sliced
- 4 pitted Kalamata olives, sliced
- 1 ½ tbsps capers, rinsed and drained

Directions

- Add quinoa, water, and salt to a medium pot and cook for 15 minutes.

- In a bowl, mix tomatoes, green olives, olives, capers, garlic, olive oil, parsley, basil, and red chili flakes.

- Allow sitting for 5 minutes. Serve the puttanesca with the quinoa.

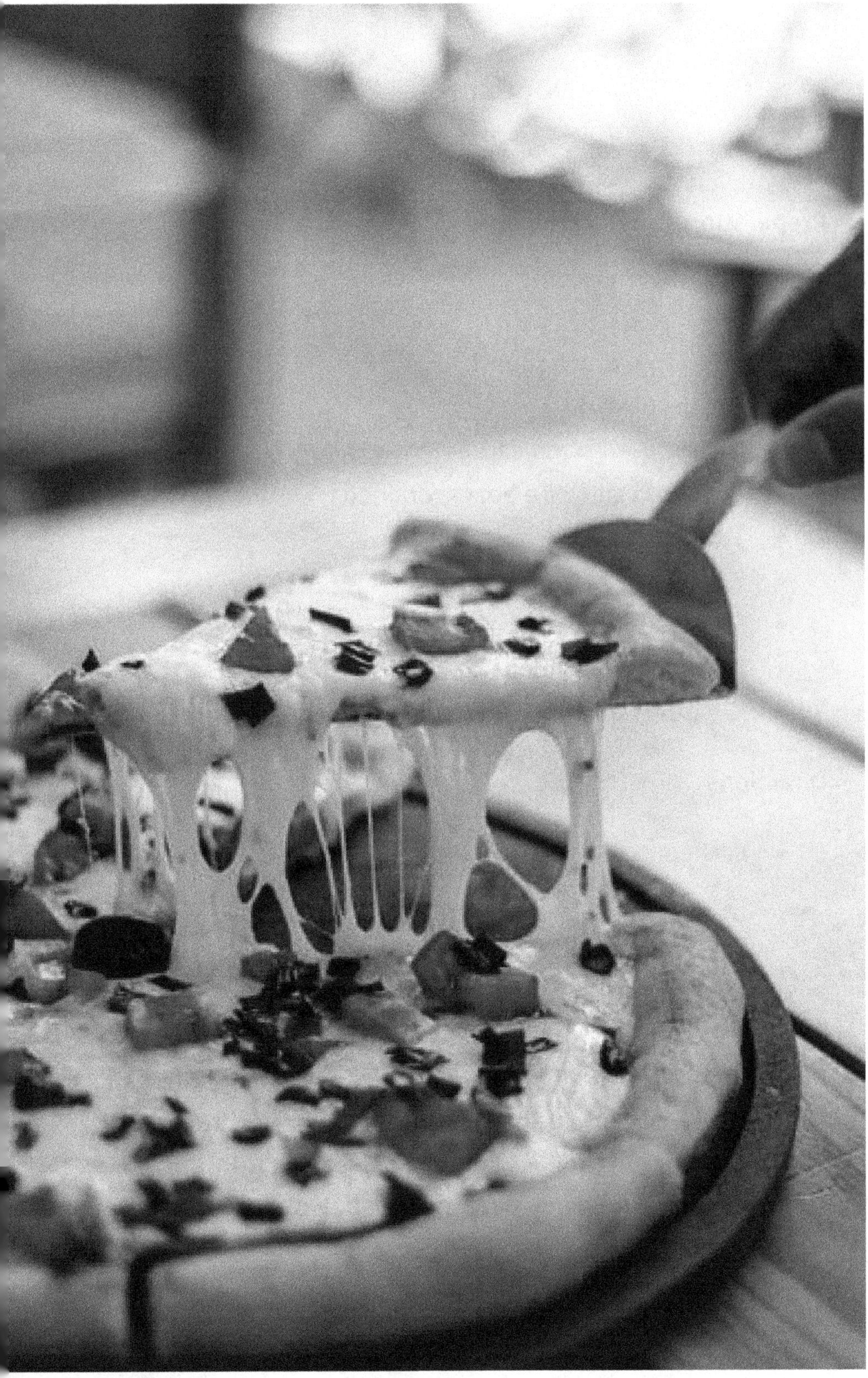

Acorn Squash Stuffed with Beans & Spinach

6 Servings

Preparation Time: 60 minutes

Ingredients

- 2 lbs large acorn squash
- 2 tbsps olive oil
- 3 garlic cloves, minced
- 1 (15 oz) can white beans, drained
- 1 cup chopped spinach leaves
- ½ cup vegetable stock
- Salt and black pepper to taste
- ½ tsp cumin powder
- ½ tsp chili powder

Directions

- Preheat the oven to 350 F.

- Cut the squash in half and scoop out the seeds. Season with salt and pepper and place face down on a sheet pan. Bake for 45 minutes.

- Heat olive oil in a pot over medium heat. Sauté garlic until fragrant, 30 seconds and mix in beans and spinach, allow wilting for 2 minutes and season with salt, black pepper, cumin powder, and chili powder.

- Cook for 2 minutes and turn the heat off. When the squash is fork-tender, remove from the oven and fill the holes with the bean and spinach mixture. Serve.

SNACKS & SIDES

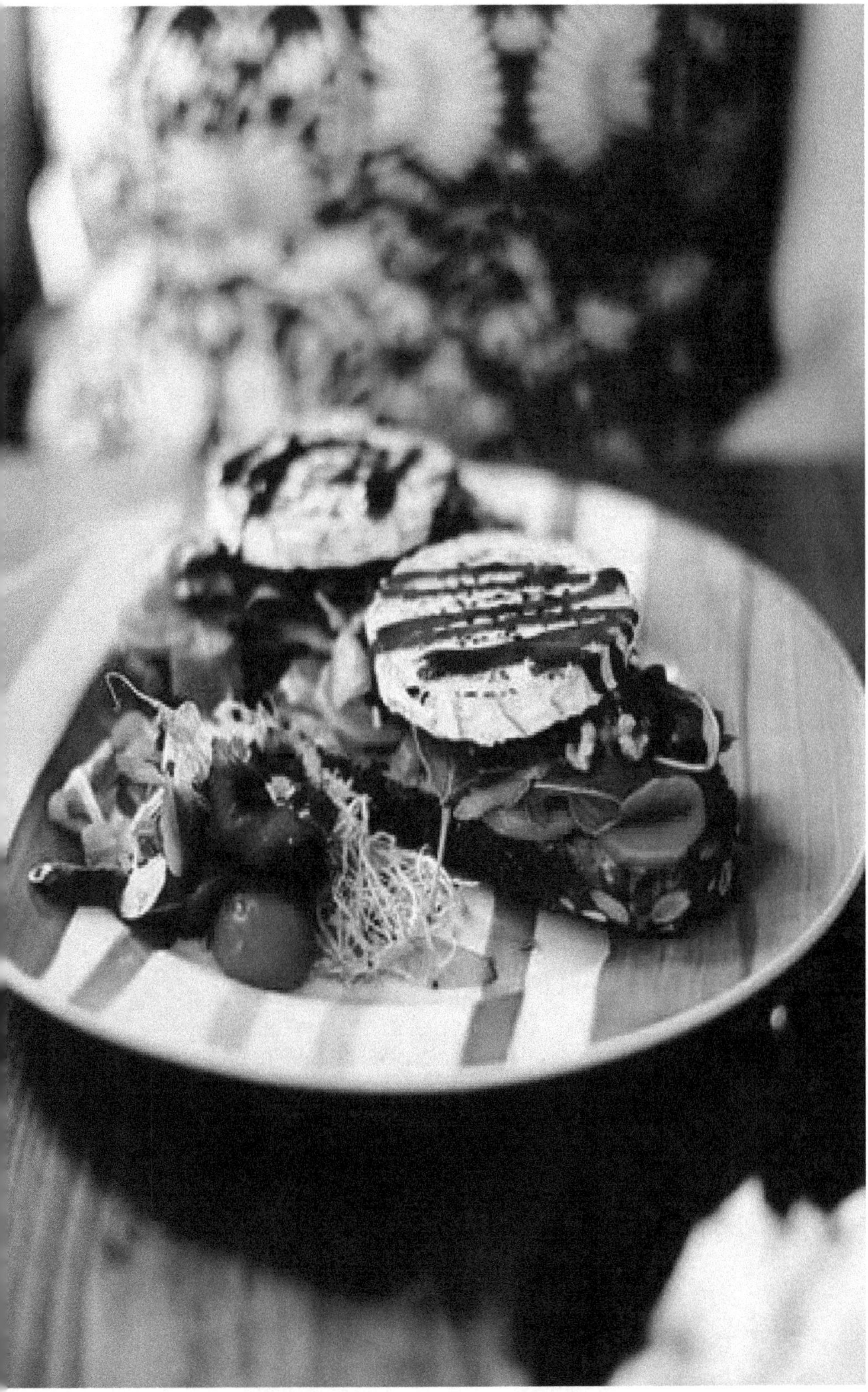

Berries, Nuts & Cream Bowl

6 Servings

Preparation time: 30 minutes

Ingredients

- 5 tbsps flaxseed powder
- 1 cup dairy-free dark chocolate
- 1 cup plant butter
- 2 tsps vanilla extract
- 2 cups fresh blueberries
- 4 tbsps lemon juice
- 2 cups coconut cream
- 4 oz walnuts, chopped
- ½ cup roasted coconut chips

Directions

- Preheat oven to 320 F.

- Grease a springform pan with cooking spray and line with parchment paper.

- In a bowl, mix the flaxseed powder with 2/3 cup water and allow thickening for 5 minutes.

- Break the chocolate and butter into a bowl and melt in the microwave for 1-2 minutes.

- Share the vegan "flax egg" into two bowls; whisk 1 pinch of salt into one portion and then 1 teaspoon of vanilla into the other.

- Pour the chocolate mixture into the vanilla mixture and combine well.

- Fold into the other vegan "flax egg" mixture.

- Pour the batter into the springform pan and bake for 15-20 minutes.

- When ready, slice the cake into squares and share it into serving bowls. Set aside.

- Pour blueberries, lemon juice, and the remaining vanilla into a bowl.

- Break blueberries and allow sitting for a few minutes.

- Whip the coconut cream with a whisk until a soft peak forms.

- Spoon the cream on the cakes, top with the blueberry mixture, and sprinkle with walnuts and coconut flakes. Serve.

Paprika Baked Beans

2 Serving

Preparation time: 30 minutes

Ingredients

- 2 (14-oz) can white beans
- 4 tbsps soy sauce
- 2 tbsps nutritional yeast
- 2 tsps smoked paprika
- 2 tsps onion powder
- 1 tsp garlic powder

Directions

- Preheat oven to 390 F.

- Mix the beans, soy sauce, yeast, paprika, onion powder, and garlic powder.

- Arrange on a greased baking sheet and bake for 20-25 minutes, turning once.

- Lower the heat and bake until dried and crispy.

- Heat the oil in a skillet over medium heat. Place the burgers and fry for 10-12 minutes on both sides.

- Spread a layer of the mustard over each bun half.

- Top the bottom buns with the lettuce, tomato, onion, avocado, and burgers and cover with the remaining bun half.

- Serve right away.

Middle Eastern Onion Phyllo

8 Servings

Preparation time: 25 minutes

Ingredients

- 2 tbsps olive oil
- 2 medium onions, thinly sliced
- 1 garlic clove, minced
- 1 tsp chopped fresh rosemary
- Salt and black pepper to taste
- 1 tbsp chopped dill pickles
- 1 sheet vegan puff pastry, thawed
- 18 pitted black olives, quartered

Directions

- Warm the oil in a skillet over medium heat.

- Place in onions, garlic, rosemary, salt, and pepper and sauté for 5 minutes.

- Add in dill pickles, stir and set aside.

- Preheat oven to 390 F.

- Roll out the pastry and, using a small bowl, cut into 3-inch circles.

- Arrange the circles on a greased baking sheet and top with onion mixture.

- Scatter the olives over. Bake for 15 minutes until golden brown.

- Serve warm.

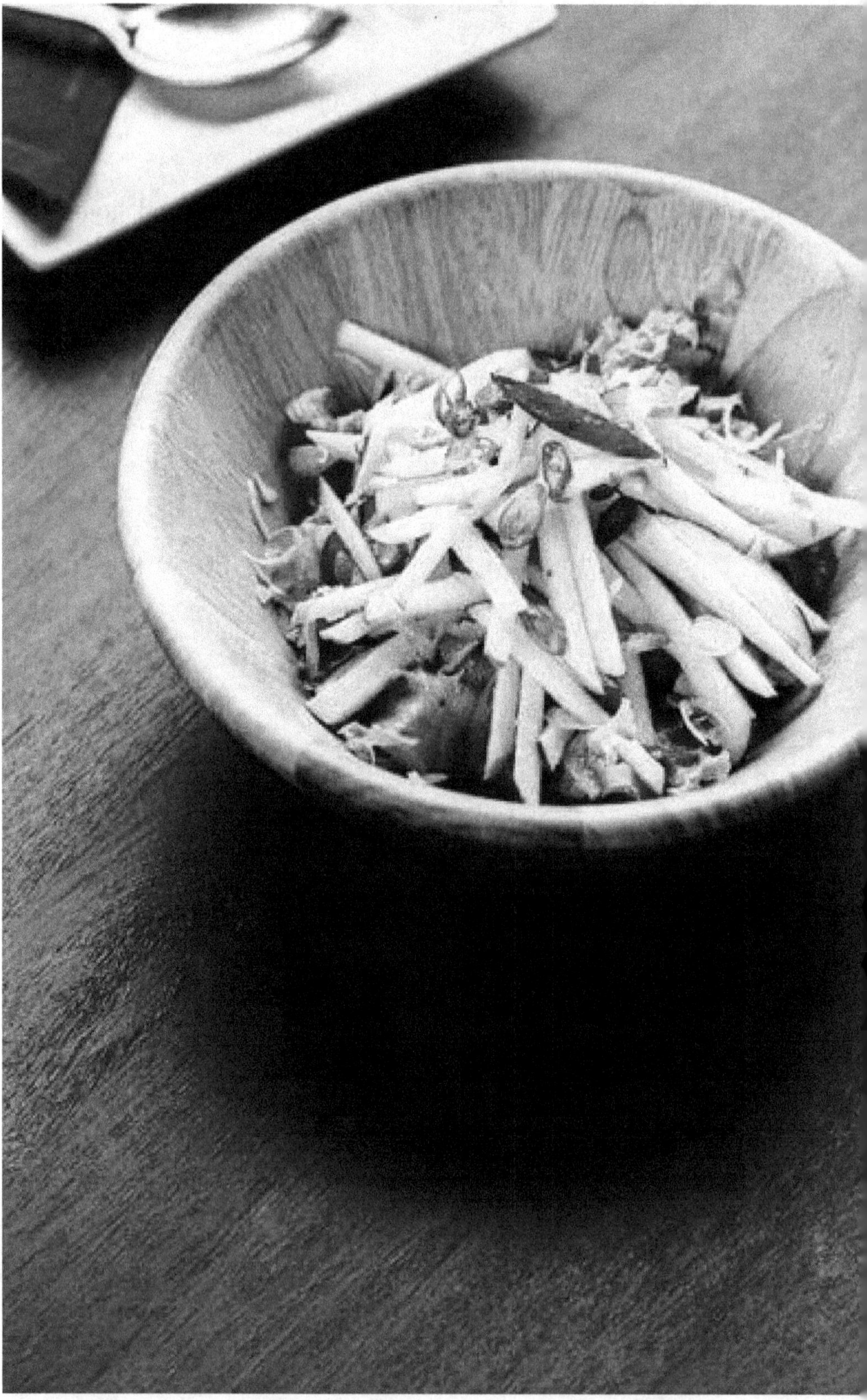

Arugula & Hummus Pitas

8 Servings

Preparation time: 15 minutes

Ingredients

- 8 pieces of whole-wheat pita bread, halved
- 2 garlic cloves, chopped
- 2 cups tahini
- 4 tbsps fresh lemon juice
- ¼ tsp ground cayenne
- ½ cup water
- 2 (15.5-oz) can chickpeas
- 4 medium carrots, grated
- 2 large ripe tomatoes, sliced
- 4 cups arugula

Directions

- In a food processor, add in garlic, tahini, lemon juice, salt, cayenne pepper, and water.

- Pulse until smooth.

- In a bowl, mash the chickpeas with a fork.

- Stir in carrots and tahini mixture; reserve.

- Spread the hummus over the pitas and top with a tomato slice and arugula.

- Serve immediately.

Authentic Guacamole

4 Servings

Preparation time: 10 minutes

Ingredients

- 4 ripe avocados
- 4 garlic cloves, pressed
- Zest and juice of 2 lime
- 2 tsps ground cumin
- 2 tomatoes, chopped
- 2 tbsps cilantro, chopped

Directions

- Place the avocados in a bowl and mash them.

- Stir in garlic, lime juice, lime zest, cumin, tomato, cilantro, salt, and pepper.

- Serve immediately.

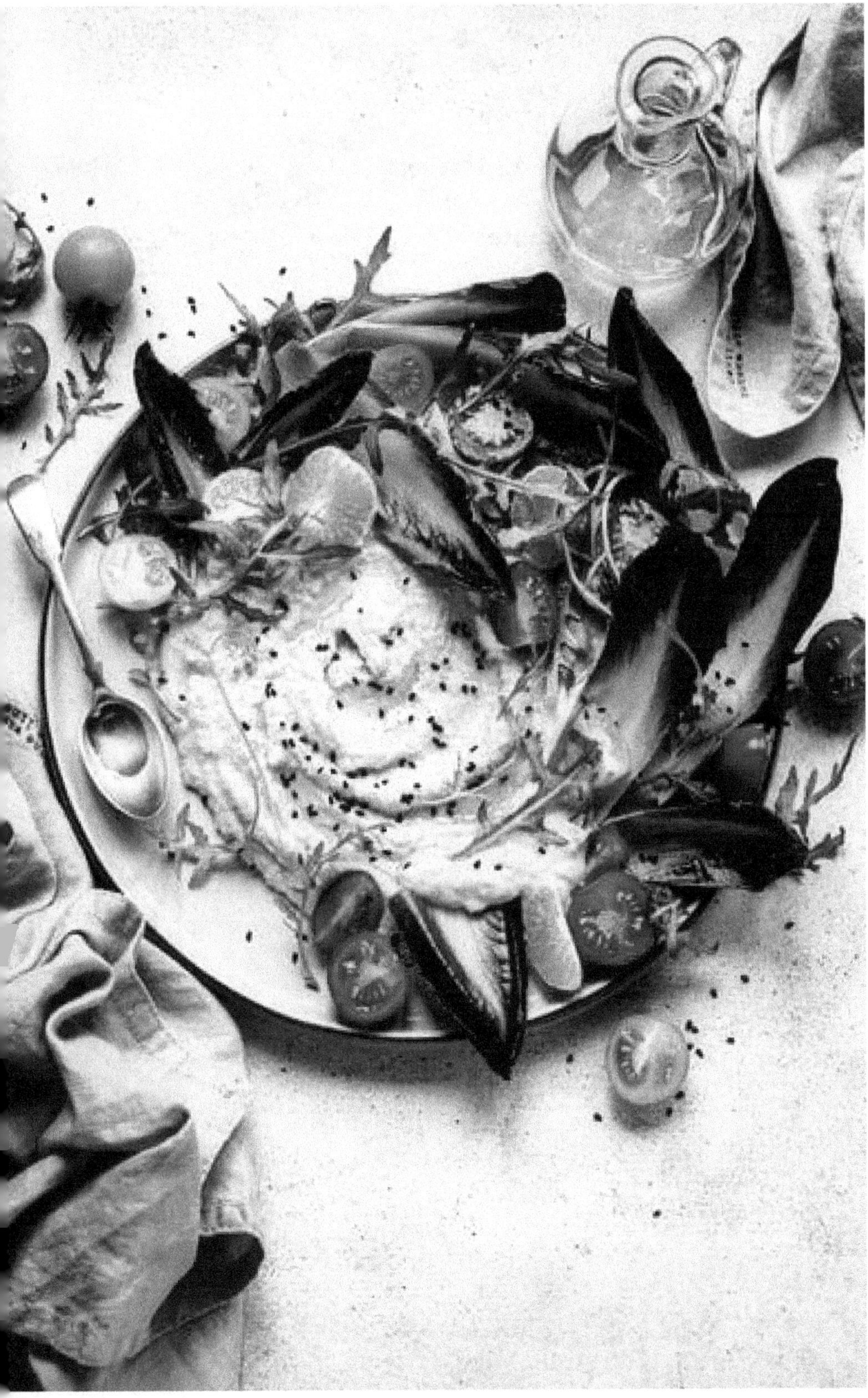

Cucumber Stuffed Tomatoes

12 Servings

Preparation time: 15 minutes

Ingredients

- 12 tomatoes, whole
- 4 cucumbers, chopped
- Juice of 12 lemon
- 1 red bell pepper, minced
- 4 green onions, finely minced
- 2 tbsps minced fresh tarragon

Directions

- Remove the tops of the tomatoes.

- Using a tablespoon, scoop out the seeds and pulp.

- Arrange them on a platter. Combine the cucumbers, lemon juice, bell pepper, scallions, tarragon, and salt in a bowl.

- Stir to combine. Divide the mixture between the tomatoes and serve.

Minty Berry Cocktail

8 Servings

Preparation time: 15 minutes

Ingredients

- 4 tbsps pineapple juice
- 2 tbsps fresh lime juice
- 2 tbsps agave nectar
- 4 tsps minced fresh mint
- 4 cups pitted fresh prunes
- 2 cups fresh blueberries
- 2 cups fresh strawberries, halved
- 1 cup fresh raspberries

Directions

- Whisk the pineapple juice, lime juice, agave nectar, and mint in a bowl.

- Set aside.

- In another bowl, combine the prunes, blueberries, strawberries, and raspberries. Pour over the dressing and toss to coat.

- Serve right away.

Swiss Chard & Pecan Stuffed Mushrooms

8 Servings

Preparation time: 20 minutes

Ingredients

- 16 oz white mushrooms, stems chopped and reserved
- 4 tbsps olive oil
- 2 garlic cloves, minced
- 2 cups cooked Swiss chard
- 2 cups finely chopped pecans
- 1 cup breadcrumbs
- Salt and black pepper to taste

Directions

- Preheat oven to 390 F.

- Warm oil in a skillet over medium heat, add the mushroom stems and garlic and sauté for 3 minutes.

- Mix in chard, pecans, breadcrumbs, salt, and pepper.

- Cook for another 2 minutes, stirring occasionally.

- Divide the resulting mixture between the mushroom caps and arrange on a greased baking dish.

- Bake for 15 minutes, until golden. Serve immediately.

Primavera Lettuce Rolls

8 Servings

Preparation time: 20 minutes

Ingredients

- 2 tbsps olive oil
- 4 oz rice noodles
- 4 tbsps Thai basil, chopped
- 2 tbsps cilantro, chopped
- 2 garlic cloves, minced
- 2 tbsps minced fresh ginger
- Juice of 1 lime
- 4 tbsps soy sauce
- 2 avocados, sliced
- 4 carrots, peeled and julienned
- 16 leaves butter lettuce

Directions

- In a bowl, place the noodles in hot water and let them sit for 4 minutes.

- Drain and mix with the olive oil. Allow cooling.

- Combine the basil, cilantro, garlic, ginger, lime juice, and soy sauce in another bowl.

- Add in cooked noodles, avocado, and carrots. Divide the mixture between the lettuce leaves. Fold in and secure with toothpicks. Serve right away.

SOUPS & SALADS

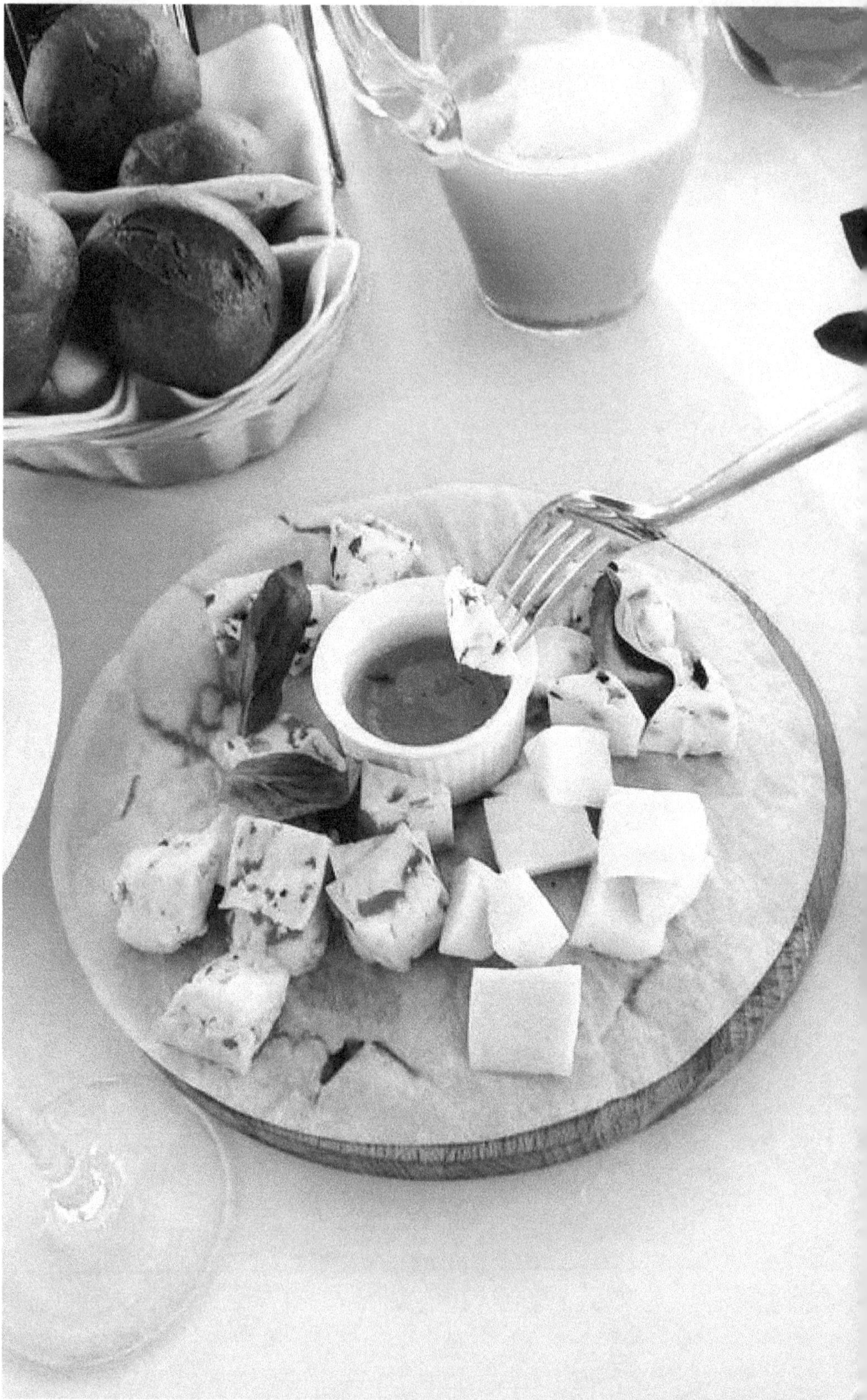

Mediterranean Soup

6 Servings

Preparation Time: 20 minutes

Ingredients

- 2 tsps Olive oil
- 1 Leek, chopped
- 4 Garlic cloves, minced
- 2 Carrots, peeled and chopped
- 1 tbsp Dried herbs
- 4 cups Vegetable broth
- 2 (15-oz) cans White beans
- 2 tbsps Lemon juice
- 2 cups Green beans

Directions

- Warm the oil in a pot over medium heat.

- Add in leek, garlic, carrots, pepper, and salt. Cook for 5 minutes until fragrant.

- Season with dried herbs. Stir in broth, green beans, and white beans, reduce the heat and simmer for 10 minutes.

- Stir in lemon juice and serve.

Vegetable and vermicelli Soup

8 Servings

Preparation Time: 20 minutes

Ingredients

- 1 tbsp Olive oil 1 onion, chopped
- 6 cups Vegetable broth
- 8 oz Vrmicelli
- 1 (5-oz) package Baby spinach
- 4 Garlic cloves, minced
- 1 (14.5-oz) can Diced tomatoes

Directions

- Heat the oil in a pot over medium heat.

- Add in onion and garlic and cook for 3 minutes.

- Stir in tomatoes, broth, salt, and pepper.

- Bring to a boil, then lower the heat and simmer for 5 minutes.

- Pour in vermicelli and spinach and cook for another 5 minutes. Serve warm.

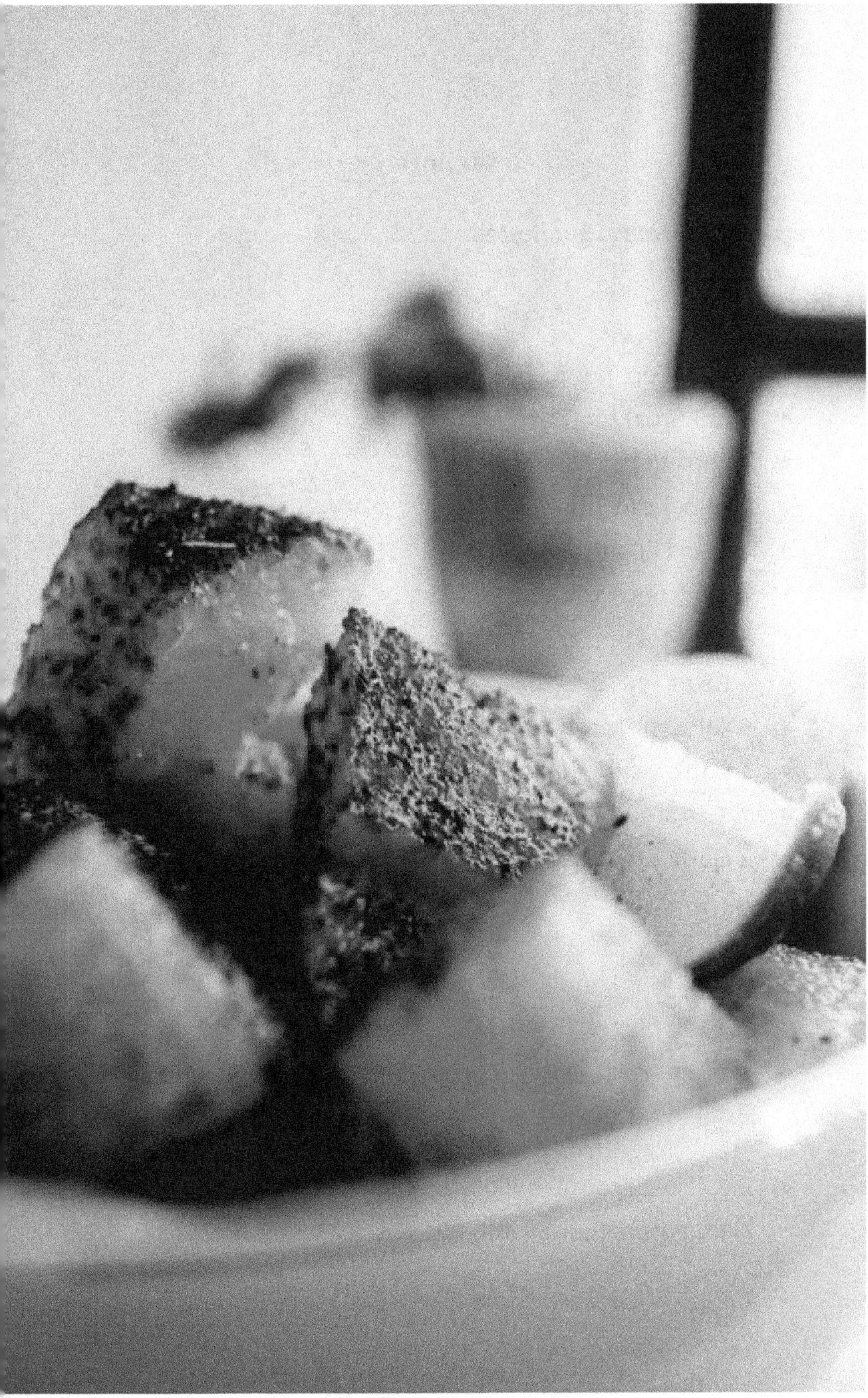

Mushroom Curry Soup

6 Servings

Preparation Time: 15 minutes

Ingredients

- 1 tbsp Coconut oil
- 1 (13.5-oz) can Coconut milk
- 4 cups Vegetable stock
- 1 (8-oz) can Tomato sauce
- 2 tbsps Cilantro, chopped
- Juice from 1 Lime
- Salt to taste
- 2 tbsps red Curry paste
- 1 red Onion, sliced
- 1 Carrot, chopped
- ½ cup sliced Shiitake mushrooms
- 2 Garlic cloves, minced

Directions

- Melt coconut oil in a pot over medium heat.

- Add in onion, garlic, carrot, and mushrooms and sauté for 5 minutes.

- Pour in coconut milk, vegetable stock, tomato sauce, cilantro, lime juice, salt, and curry paste.

- Cook until heated through. Serve.

Garlicky Broccoli Soup

8 Servings

Preparation Time: 35 minutes

Ingredients

- 2 tbsps Olive oil
- 2 cups Broccoli florets, chopped
- 2 Garlic cloves, minced
- 1 cup plain unsweetened Soy milk
- Salt and Black pepper to taste
- 1 tbsp minced Chives
- 3 spring Onions, chopped
- 6 cups Vegetable broth
- 3 Potatoes, chopped

Directions

- Warm the oil in a pot over medium heat.

- Add in spring onions and garlic and sauté for 5 minutes until translucent.

- Add in broth, potatoes, and broccoli. Bring to a boil, then lower the heat and simmer for 20 minutes.

- Mix in soy milk, salt, and pepper. Cook for 5 more minutes. Serve topped with chives.

Vegetable & Black Bean Soup

6 Servings

Preparation Time: 50 minutes

Ingredients

- 2 tbsps Olive oil
- 2 Garlic cloves, minced
- 2 Tomatoes, chopped
- 4 cups Vegetable broth
- 1 (15.5-oz) can Black beans
- 1 tsp dried thyme
- ¼ tsp Cayenne pepper
- 1 tbsp Minced cilantro
- 1 Onion, chopped
- 1 Celery stalk, chopped
- 2 medium Carrots, chopped
- 1 small Green bell pepper, chopped

Directions

- Warm the oil in a pot over medium heat.

- Add in onion, celery, carrots, bell pepper, garlic, and tomatoes. Sauté for 5 minutes, stirring often.

- Add in broth, beans, thyme, salt, and cayenne.

- Bring to a boil, then lower the heat and simmer for 15 minutes.

- Transfer the soup to a food processor and pulse until smooth.

- Serve in soup bowls garnished with cilantro.

Tangy Nutty Brussel Sprout Salad

6 Servings

Preparation Time: 20 minutes

Ingredients

- 1 lb Brussels sprouts, grated
- 1 tsp Chili paste
- 2 oz Pecans
- 1 oz Pumpkin seeds
- 1 oz Sunflower seeds
- ½ tsp Cumin powder
- 1 Lemon, juiced and zested
- ½ cup Olive oil
- 1 tbsp Plant butter

Directions

- Put Brussels sprouts in a salad bowl.

- In a small bowl, mix lemon juice, zest, olive oil, salt, and pepper, and drizzle the dressing over the Brussels sprouts.

- Toss and allow the vegetable to marinate for 10 minutes.

- Melt plant butter in a pan.

- Stir in chili paste and toss the pecans, pumpkin seeds, sunflower seeds, cumin powder, and salt in the chili butter.

- Sauté on low heat for 3-4 minutes just to heat the nuts. Allow cooling.

- Pour the nuts and seeds mix in the salad bowl, toss, and serve.

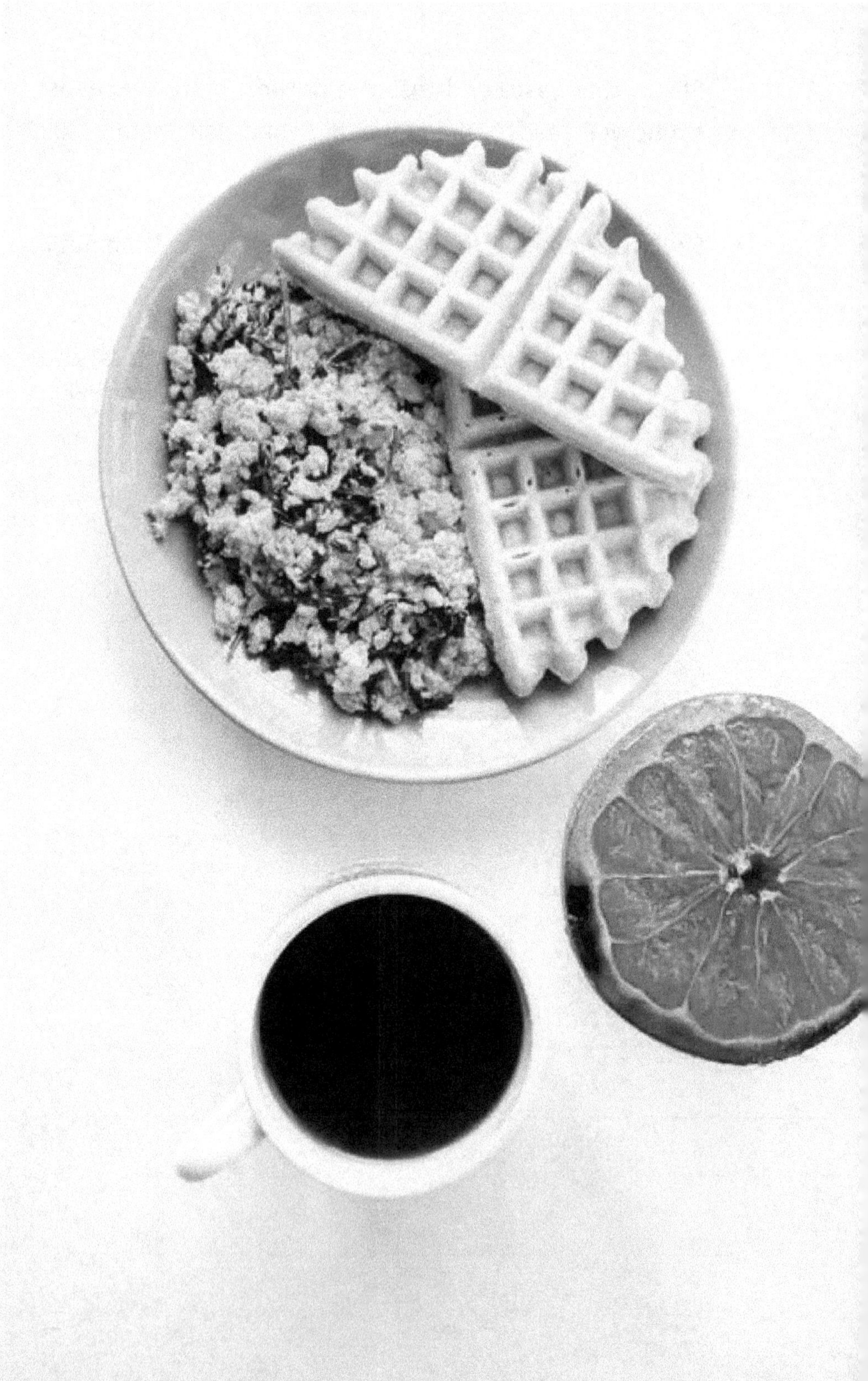

Warm Collard Salad

4 Servings

Preparation Time: 10 minutes

Ingredients

- ¾ cup Coconut whipping cream
- 1 Garlic clove, minced
- Salt and Black pepper to taste
- 2 oz Plant butter
- 1 cup Collards, rinsed
- 4 oz Tofu cheese
- 2 tbsps Tofu mayonnaise
- A pinch of Mustard powder
- 2 tbsps Coconut oil

Directions

- In a small bowl, whisk the coconut whipping cream, tofu mayonnaise, mustard powder, coconut oil, garlic, salt, and black pepper until well mixed; set aside.

- Melt the plant butter in a large pan over medium heat and sauté the collards until wilted and brownish.

- Season with salt and black pepper to taste.

- Transfer the collards to a salad bowl and pour the creamy dressing over.

- Mix the salad well and crumble the tofu cheese over. Serve.

Bean & Couscous Salad

6 Servings

Preparation Time: 15 minutes

Ingredients

- ¼ cup Olive oil
- 1 yellow Bell pepper, chopped
- 1 Carrot, shredded
- ½ cup chopped dried Apricots
- ¼ cup Golden raisins
- ¼ cup chopped Roasted cashews
- 1 (15.5-oz) can White beans
- 2 tbsps minced fresh Cilantro leaves
- 2 tbsps fresh Lemon juice
- 1 medium Shallot, minced
- ½ tsp ground Coriander
- ½ tsp Turmeric
- ¼ tsp ground Cayenne
- 1 cup Couscous
- 2 cups Vegetable broth

Directions

- Warm 1 tbsp of oil in a pot over medium heat.

- Place in shallot, coriander, turmeric, cayenne pepper, and couscous. Cook for 2 minutes, stirring often.

- Add in broth and salt. Bring to a boil.

- Turn the heat off and let sit covered for 5 minutes.

- Remove to a bowl and stir in bell pepper, carrot, apricots, raisins, cashews, beans, and cilantro. Set aside.

- In another bowl, whisk the remaining oil with lemon juice until blended.

- Pour over the salad and toss to combine. Serve immediately.

DINNER

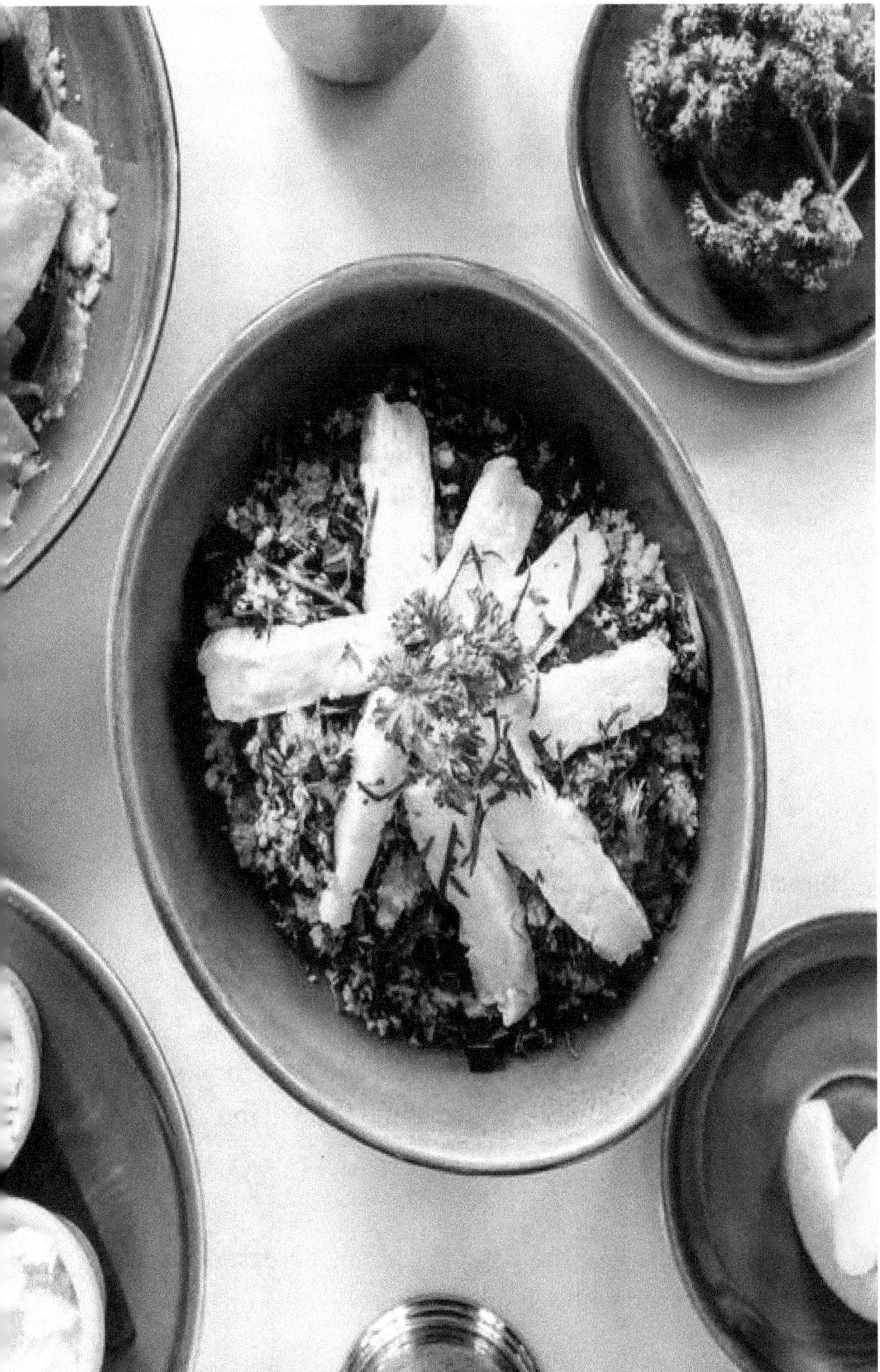

Baked Potatoes & Asparagus & Pine Nuts

8 Servings

Preparation time: 50 minutes

Ingredients

- 2 bunch of asparagus, sliced
- 4 tbsps olive oil
- 4 garlic cloves, minced
- 10 cups fresh baby spinach
- Salt and black pepper to taste
- 2 tsps dried basil
- 1 tsp dried thyme
- 4 potatoes, sliced
- 1 cup vegetable broth
- 4 tbsps nutritional yeast
- 1 cup ground pine nuts

Directions

- Heat oven to 370 F.

- Heat half of the oil in a skillet over medium heat. Put in garlic, spinach, salt, and pepper and heat for 4 minutes until the spinach wilts. Add in basil and thyme.

- Set aside.

- Arrange half of the potato slices on a greased casserole and season with salt and pepper.

- Top with the asparagus slices and finish with the spinach mixture.

- Cover with the remaining potato slices.

- Whisk the broth with nutritional yeast in a bowl.

- Put in some of the vegetables.

- Sprinkle with remaining oil and pine nuts. Cover with foil and bake for 40 minutes.

- Uncover and bake for another 10 minutes until golden brown. Serve warm.

Italian Potato & Swiss Chard Au Gratin

4 Servings

Preparation time: 1 hour 15 minutes

Ingredients

- 6 tbsps olive oil
- 2 medium yellow onions, minced
- 6 garlic cloves, minced
- 2 cups Swiss chard, chopped
- Salt and black pepper to taste
- 4 lbs new potatoes, unpeeled, sliced
- 2 tsps Italian seasoning
- 4 tbsps plant-based Parmesan

Directions

- Heat the oven to 360 F.

- Heat half of the oil in a skillet over medium heat.

- Place in onion and garlic and sauté for 3 minutes until translucent.

- Add in Swiss chard to wilt for 3-4 minutes. Season with salt and pepper.

- Set aside.

- Arrange half of the potato slices on a greased baking dish.

- Sprinkle with Italian seasoning, salt, and pepper.

- Sprinkle with the remaining olive oil. Top with Swiss chard mixture and cover with the remaining potatoes.

- Cover with foil and bake for 1 hour.

- Scatter Parmesan cheese over and bake for another 10 minutes. Serve immediately.

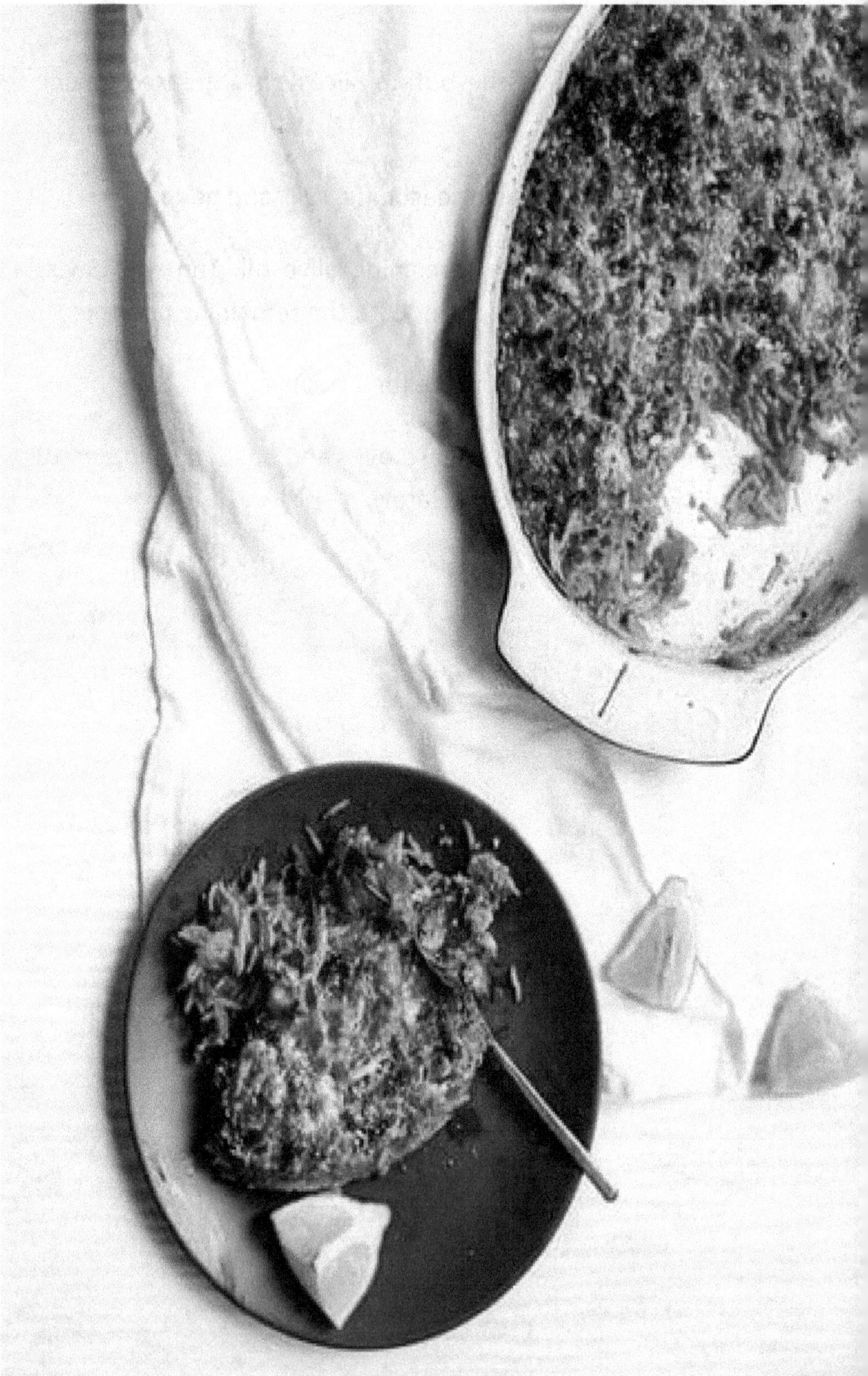

Bean & Pecan Stuffed Mushrooms

8 Servings

Preparation time: 45 minutes

Ingredients

- 8 mushroom caps
- 4 tbsps olive oil
- 2 onions, minced
- 4 garlic cloves, minced
- 2 carrots, chopped
- 2 (15.5-oz) can white beans, mashed
- 2 cups finely chopped pecans
- 4 tbsps minced fresh parsley
- 1 cup dry breadcrumbs

Directions

- Preheat oven to 360 F.

- Heat the oil in a skillet over medium temperature.

- Put the onion, garlic, and carrot and sauté for 5 minutes until tender.

- Put in beans, pecans, parsley, and half of the breadcrumbs. Sprinkle with salt and pepper.

- Stuff the mushrooms with the mixture and arrange on a greased baking dish.

- Cover with baking foil and bake for 20 minutes.

- Uncover and scatter with the remaining breadcrumbs.

- Bake another 10 minutes until golden brown. Serve warm.

French Vegetable Byaldi

12 Servings

Preparation time: 75 minutes

Ingredients

- 4 potatoes, sliced
- 4 eggplants, sliced diagonally
- 6 tbsps olive oil
- 2 onions, chopped
- 6 garlic cloves, minced
- 6 cups spinach, chopped
- 4 cups kale, chopped
- 4 cups collard greens, chopped
- 2 cups loosely packed basil leaves
- 12 ripe plum tomatoes, sliced
- 2 ¼ cup breadcrumbs
- 6 tbsps plant-based Parmesan

Directions

- Heat the oven to 390 F.

- Put the potato slices on a greased baking sheet and the eggplant slices in a separate baking sheet.

- Sprinkle the vegetables with salt, oil and pepper.

- Bake the eggplants for 10 minutes and the potato for 20 minutes. Set aside.

- Heat the oil in a pot over medium temperature.

- Put in onion and garlic and sauté for 3 minutes until soft.

- Add in spinach, kale, collard greens, salt, and pepper.

- Heat for 7 minutes until the greens wilt.

- Put the mixture to a blender.

- Add in basil and remaining oil, salt, and pepper and blend until smooth.

- On a grease baking dish, arrange half of the potato slices and cover with some greens mixture.

- Then add a layer of eggplant slices and cover with more greens mixture.

- Then add a layer of tomato slices and cover with more greens mixture. Repeat the process until any ingredients left.

- Sprinkle each layer with salt and pepper. Finally, scatter with breadcrumbs and Parmesan cheese.

- Sprinkle the remaining oil. Bake for another 10 minutes. Serve warm.

Balsamic Artichoke Hearts

8 Servings

Preparation time: 30 minutes

Ingredients

- 3 lbs artichoke hearts
- 4 tbsps olive oil
- Sea salt and black pepper to taste
- 1 cup balsamic vinegar
- Juice and zest of 2 lemon

Directions

- Preheat oven to 360 F.
- Brush the artichoke hearts with olive oil, salt, and pepper.
- Arrange on a baking sheet.
- Roast for 20-25 minutes, turning once.
- Meanwhile, put the vinegar in a skillet over medium heat and bring to a boil.
- Lower the heat and simmer for 8 minutes until it gets a syrupy texture.
- Once the artichokes are ready, coat them with lemon juice and lemon zest.
- Serve topped with balsamic reduction.

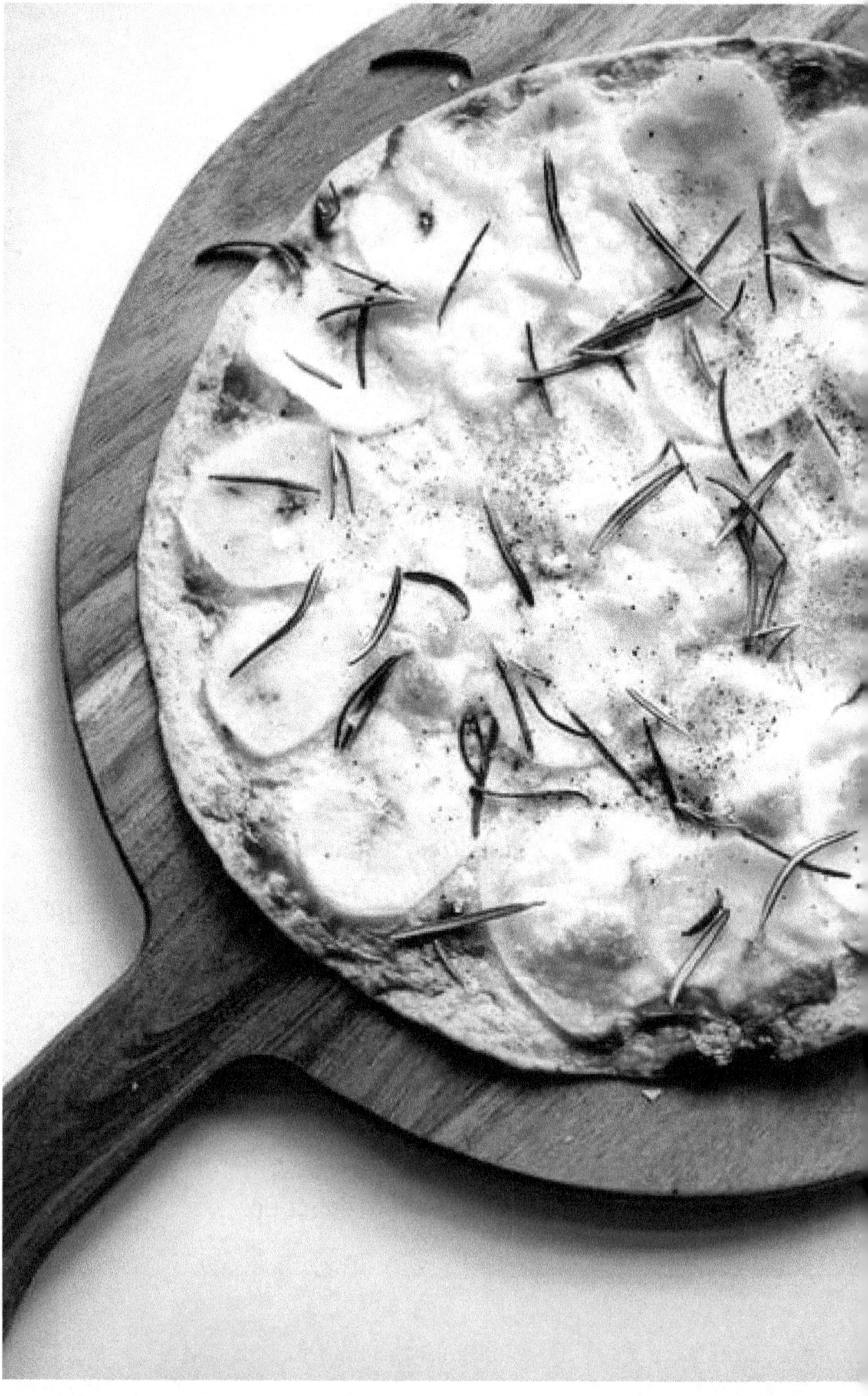

Melon & Cucumber Gazpacho

8 Servings

Preparation time: 10 minutes

Ingredients

- 4 large tomatoes
- 2 jalapeño peppers, seeded
- 8 cups cubed fresh melon, divided
- 4 tsps rice vinegar
- ½ cup extra-virgin olive oil
- 2 large cucumbers, peeled, chopped
- 2 small red onions, chopped
- 2 small red bell peppers, chopped
- ¼ cup minced fresh dill

Directions

- Put the tomatoes, jalapeño pepper, vinegar, olive oil, and half of the melon in a food processor and blitz.

- Place in cucumber, onion, bell pepper, and dill and blend until uniform and smooth.

- Adjust seasoning with salt and pepper.

- Place the remaining melon in a bowl and top with the gazpacho.

Artichoke & Tomato Tart with Peanuts

8 Servings

Preparation time: 35 minutes

Ingredients

- 2 (10-oz) package artichoke hearts
- 2 frozen puff pastry sheet, thawed
- 1 cup toasted peanuts
- 16 oz extra-firm tofu, crumbled
- 4 green onions, minced
- 4 tsps fresh lemon juice
- 4 tbsps minced fresh parsley
- 2 tbsps minced fresh marjoram
- 42 tomatoes, sliced

Directions

- Preheat oven to 390 F.

- Boil salted water in a pot over high heat.

- Place in artichoke hearts and cook for 12 minutes.

- Drain and set aside. Lay the pastry on a floured flat surface and roll out.

- Transfer to a tart dish and trim the edges. Bake for 10 minutes. Set aside.

- Cut finely 2 artichoke hearts and set aside.

- In a blender, place the remaining hearts, half of the peanuts, tofu, and green onions and pulse until finely chopped.

- Add lemon juice, parsley, marjoram, salt, and pepper.

- Blitz until smooth. Remove to a bowl and mix in remaining peanuts and reserved artichokes.

- Spread the mixture over the tart pastry and top with tomato slices. Sprinkle with salt and pepper.

- Bake for 25 minutes until golden brown. Let cool 10-15 minutes before slicing.

Chili Broccoli & Beans with Almonds

8 Servings

Preparation time: 30 minutes

Ingredients

- 3 lbs potatoes

- 8 cups broccoli florets
- 6 tbsps olive oil
- 6 garlic cloves, minced
- 2 cups chopped almonds
- ½ tsp crushed red pepper
- 2 (15.5-oz) can white beans
- 2 tsps dried thyme
- 2 tbsps fresh lemon juice

Directions

- Place the potatoes in water and cook for 20 minutes. Set aside.

- Place the broccoli in water and steam for 7 minutes.

- Heat 2 tbsps of oil in a skillet over medium heat. Place in garlic, almonds, and red pepper and cook for 1 minute.

- Add in potatoes, broccoli, beans, thyme, salt, and pepper.

- Cook for 5 minutes. Drizzle with lemon juice and remaining oil. Serve.

DESSERTS

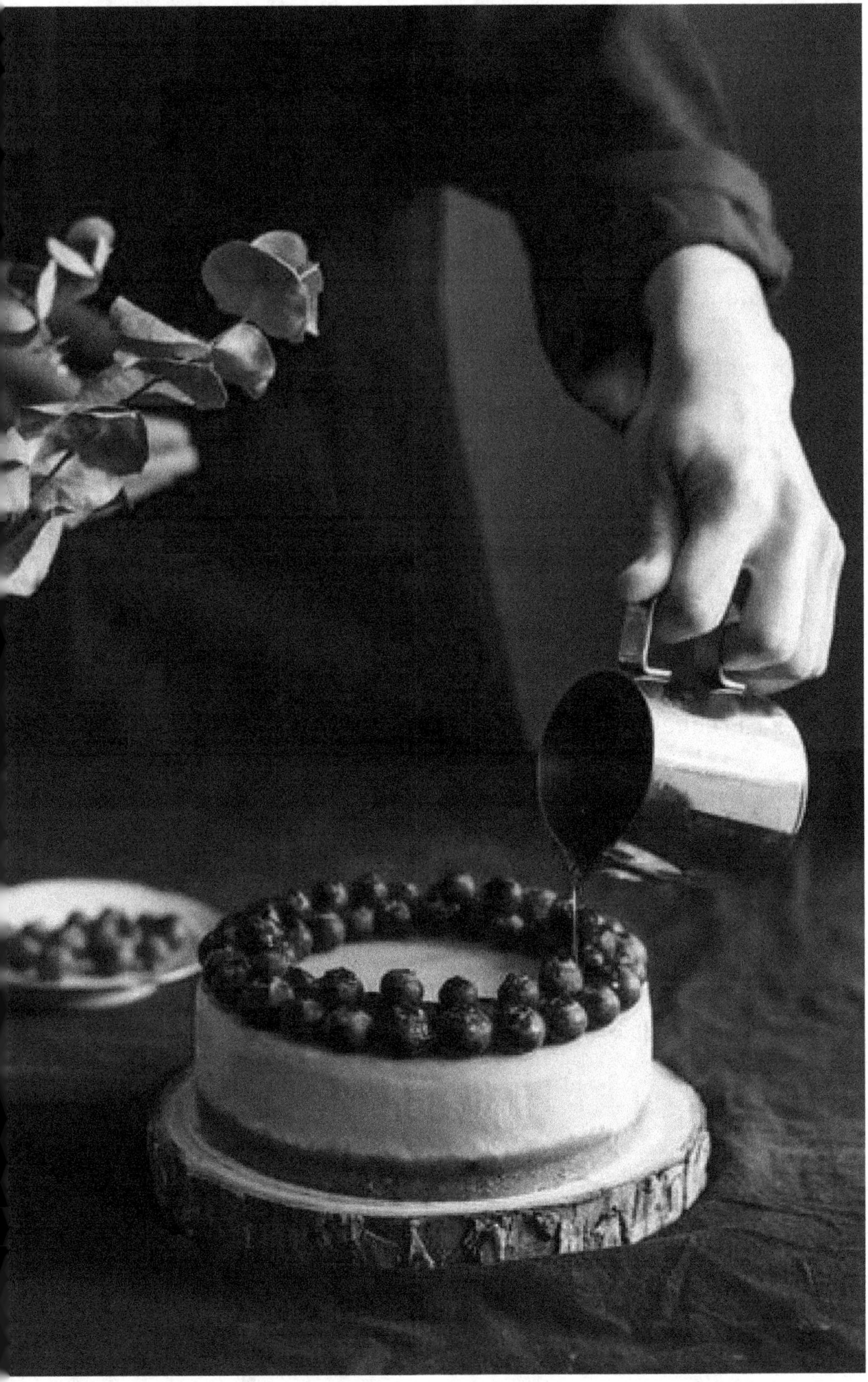

Maple Fruit Crumble

4 Servings

Preparation time: 30 minutes

Ingredients

- 3 cups chopped apricots
- 3 cups chopped mangoes
- 4 tbsps pure maple syrup
- 1 cup gluten-free rolled oats
- ½ cup shredded coconut
- 2 tbsps coconut oil

Directions

- Preheat oven to 360 F.

- Place the apricots, mangoes, and 2 tbsps of maple syrup in a round baking dish.

- In a food processor, put the oats, coconut, coconut oil, and remaining maple syrup. Blend until combined. Pour over the fruit. Bake for 20-25 minutes. Allow cooling before slicing and serving.

Sherry-Lime Mango Dessert

4 Servings

Preparation time: 15 minutes

Ingredients

- 3 ripe mangoes, cubed
- ⅓ cup pure date sugar
- 2 tbsps fresh lime juice
- ½ cup Sherry wine
- Fresh mint sprigs

Directions

- Arrange the mango cubes on a baking sheet. Sprinkle with some dates and let sit covered for 30 minutes.

- Sprinkle with lime juice and sherry wine. Refrigerate covered for 1 hour. Remove from the fridge and let sit for a few minutes at room temperature.

- Serve in glasses topped with mint.

Almond & Chia Bites with Cherries

2 Servings

Preparation time: 30 minutes

Ingredients

- 1 cup cherries, pitted
- 1 cup shredded coconut
- ¼ cup chia seeds
- ¾ cup ground almonds
- ¼ cup cocoa nibs

Directions

- Blend cherries, coconut, chia seeds, almonds, and cocoa nibs in a food processor until crumbly.

- Shape the mixture into 24 balls and arrange on a lined baking sheet. Let sit in the fridge for 15 minutes.

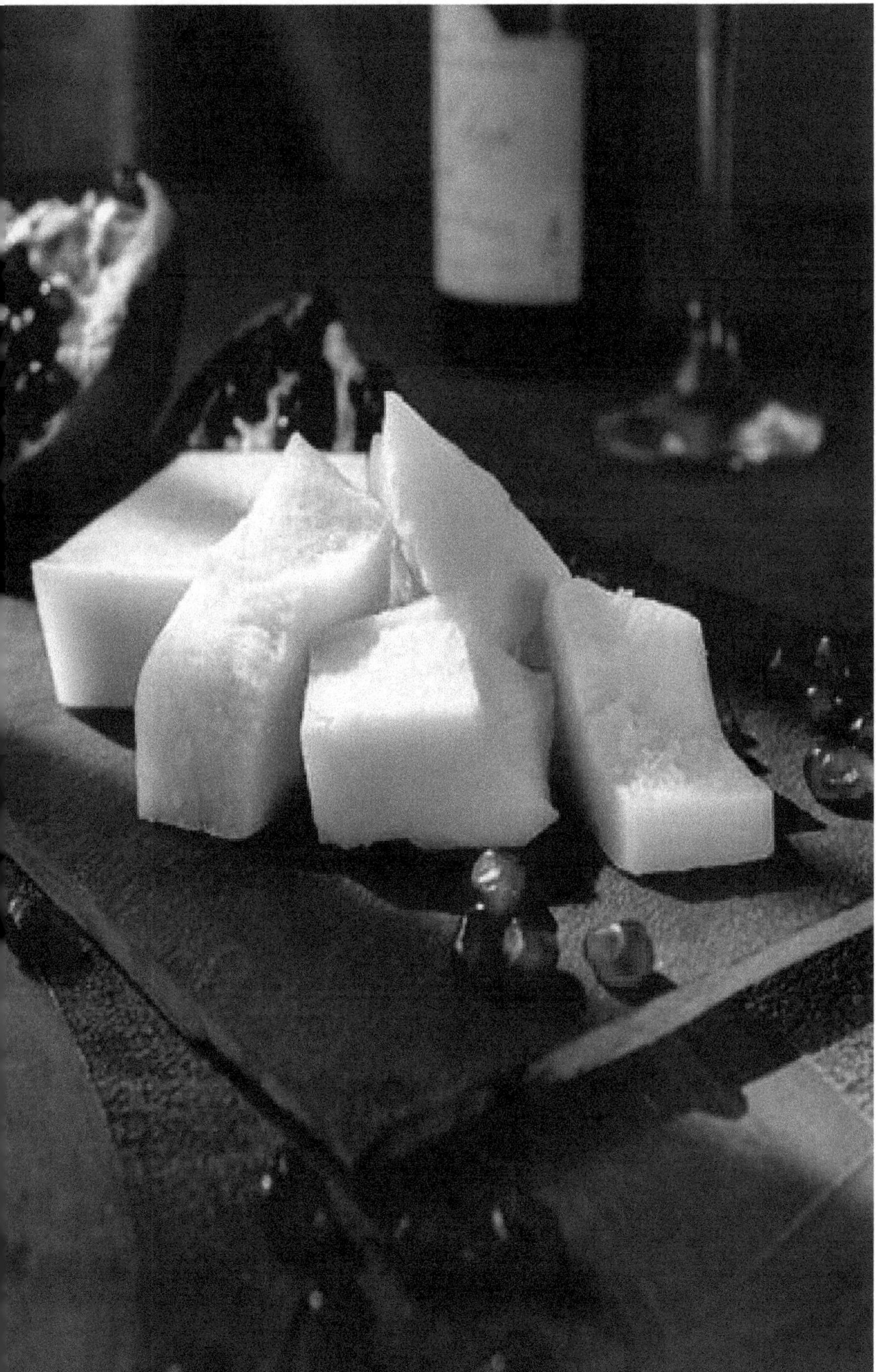

Glazed Chili Chocolate Cake

4 Servings

Preparation time: 40 minutes

Ingredients

- 1 ¾ cups whole-grain flour
- 1 cup pure date sugar
- ¼ cup unsweetened cocoa powder
- 1 tsp baking soda
- ½ tsp baking powder
- 1 ½ tsps ground cinnamon
- ¼ tsp ground chili
- ⅓ cup olive oil
- 1 tbsp apple cider vinegar
- 1 ½ tsps pure vanilla extract
- 2 (1-oz) squares vegan chocolate
- ¼ cup soy milk
- ½ cup pure date sugar
- 3 tbsps plant butter
- ½ tsp pure vanilla extract

Directions

- Preheat oven to 360 F.

- In a bowl, mix the flour, sugar, baking soda, baking powder, cinnamon, and chili.

- In another bowl, whisk the oil, vinegar, vanilla, and 1 cup cold water. Pour into the flour mixture, stir to combine. Pour the batter into a greased baking pan. Bake for 30 minutes. Let cool for 10-15 minutes. Take out the cake inverted onto a wire rack and allow to cool completely.

- Place the chocolate and soy milk in a pot. Cook until the chocolate is melted. Add in sugar, cook for 5 minutes. Turn the heat off and mix in butter and vanilla. Cover the cake with the glaze. Refrigerate until the glaze is set. Serve.

Vanilla Cranberry & Almond Balls

12 Servings

Preparation time: 30 minutes

Ingredients

- 2 tbsps almond butter
- 2 tbsps maple syrup
- ¾ cup cooked millet
- ¼ cup sesame seeds, toasted
- 1 tbsp chia seeds
- ½ tsp almond extract
- Zest of 1 orange
- 1 tbsp dried cranberries
- ¼ cup ground almonds

Directions

- Whisk the almond butter and syrup in a bowl until creamy. Mix in millet, sesame seeds, chia seeds, almond extract, orange zest, cranberries, and almonds.

- Shape the mixture into balls and arrange on a parchment paper-lined baking sheet. Let chill in the fridge for 15 minutes.

Pressure Cooker Apple Cupcakes

4 Servings

Preparation time: 30 minutes

Ingredients

- 1 cup canned applesauce
- 1 cup non-dairy milk
- 6 tbsps maple syrup + for sprinkling
- ¼ cup spelt flour
- ½ tsp apple pie spice
- A pinch of salt

Directions

- In a bowl, combine the applesauce, milk, maple syrup, flour, apple pie spice, and salt. Scoop into 4 heat-proof ramekins. Drizzle with more syrup.

- Pour 1 cup of water into the pressure cooker and fit in a trivet. Place the ramekins on the trivet. Lock lid in place; set the time to 6 minutes on High. Once ready, perform a quick pressure release.

- Unlock the lid and let cool for a few minutes; take out the ramekins. Allow cooling for 10 minutes and serve.

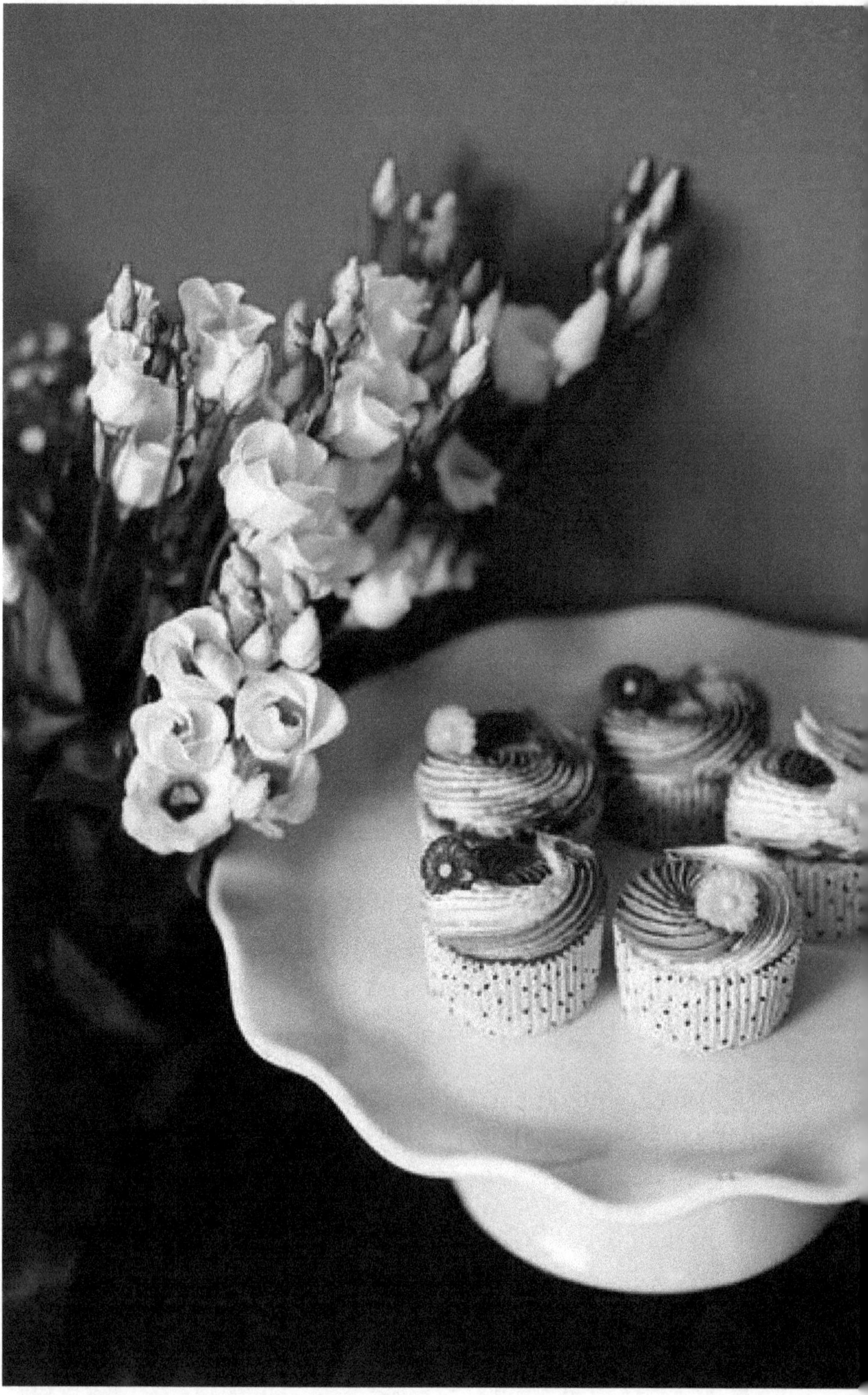

Roasted Apples Stuffed with Pecans & Dates

4 Servings

Preparation time: 40 minutes

Ingredients

- 4 apples, cored, halved lengthwise
- ½ cup finely chopped pecans
- 4 dates, pitted and chopped
- 1 tbsp plant butter
- 1 tbsp pure maple syrup
- ¼ tsp ground cinnamon

Directions

- Preheat oven to 360 F.

- Mix the pecans, dates, butter, maple syrup, and cinnamon in a bowl. Arrange the apple on a greased baking pan and fill them with the pecan mixture.

- Pour 1 tbsp of water into the baking pan. Bake for 30-40 minutes, until soft and lightly browned. Serve immediately.

CPSIA information can be obtained
at www.ICGtesting.com
Printed in the USA
BVHW091658120521
607126BV00006B/772